Negotiating family responsibilities

Negotiating Family Responsibilities provides a major new insight into contemporary family life, particularly kin relationships outside the nuclear family. While many people believe that the real meaning of 'family' has shrunk to the nuclear family household, there is considerable evidence to suggest that relationships with the wider kin group remain an important part of most people's lives.

Based on the findings of a major study of kinship, and including lively verbatim accounts of conversations with family members, concepts of responsibility and obligation within family life are examined. The authors expand theories on the nature of assistance within families, and argue that it is negotiated over time rather than given automatically.

Of interest to lecturers and students of social policy, anthropology, sociology and gender studies, *Negotiating Family Responsibilities* is also of considerable relevance to those seeking to understand contemporary family life, especially policy makers and those who work in the caring professions.

Janet Finch is Professor of Social Relations and **Jennifer Mason** is Lecturer in Applied Social Science, both at Lancaster University.

Negotiating family responsibilities

Janet Finch and Jennifer Mason

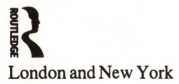

London and New York

First published in 1993
by Routledge
2 Park Square, Milton Park, Abingdon, Oxon, OX14 4RN

Simultaneously published in the USA and Canada by Routledge
a division of Routledge, Taylor & Francis
270 Madison Ave, New York NY 10016

Transferred to Digital Printing 2006

British Library Cataloguing in Publication Data
A catalogue record for this book is available from the British
Library.

Library of Congress Cataloging in Publication Data
Finch, Janet.
  Negotiating Family Responsibilities / Janet Finch
  and Jennifer Mason.
  p. cm.
  Includes bibliographical references and index.
  1. Family policy – Great Britain. 2. Family services –
  Great Britain. 3. Kinship – Great Britain.
  I. Mason, Jennifer, 1958–   . II. Title.
  HV700.G7F49   1992   92–7058
  362.82'0941 – dc20   CIP

ISBN 0–415–08406–7 (hbk)
     0–415–08407–5 (pbk)

Publisher's Note
The publisher has gone to great lengths to ensure the quality of this reprint
but points out that some imperfections in the original may be apparent

Contents

Tables

Acknowledgements

This book is based on a research study funded by ESRC grant number GOO232197, between 1985 and 1989. We are grateful for the Council's support. We would also like to thank all of the people who took part in our study as interviewees, both in the survey, and in the qualitative study. We are very grateful to them for giving us their time, their views and their experiences. Our study would not have been possible without them.

The fieldwork for the Family Obligations Survey, which formed part of the project, was undertaken by Social and Community Planning Research. We particularly appreciated the advice and support of Gill Courtenay, which ensured that the data collected were of good quality. In relation to the analysis of the survey data, we would like to acknowledge the support of Mick Green, of the Department of Applied Statistics at Lancaster University, who acted as our statistical adviser. We are very grateful for his interest in the project, and his input to it.

Our qualitative interviews were fully transcribed and analysed on a micro-computer. Secretarial and administrative support were vital to the success of the enterprise and we were very fortunate in having Nichola Hetherington with us throughout the project. She assisted us in a variety of ways with administrative tasks, in transcribing tapes and also in data analysis. Above all her interest in and enthusiasm for the project kept us on our toes and helped us to focus on issues which were important in our data. She was very ably assisted by Janet Hartley and Sandra Irving, who gave us secretarial help at different stages of the project. We would like to record our warm thanks to all of them.

There are a number of other people who helped us in various ways in our research. In this connection we would like to thank Mohammed Atcha, Hilary Conway, Ram Kaushal and Veronica Holmes. Also we received feedback on our developing analysis through papers given in a number of departments and institutions, and in particular we would like to thank colleagues in: the Department of Applied Social Science, University of Lancaster; the Centre for Women's Studies, University of Lancaster; the Social Policy Research Unit, University of York; the Department of Sociology, University of Essex; the Departments of Sociology and of Anthropology, University of Manchester; the Department of Sociology, University of Liverpool; the Faculty of Social Work, University of Toronto; the Departments of Sociology and Social Work, University of New South Wales; the Australian Institute for Family Studies; the Department of Sociology, University of Bergen; the Institute for Social Research, Oslo; the School of Nursing, University of California (San Francisco). We owe a special debt of thanks to the the Department of Social Policy and Social Work, University of Manchester, and to Professor Paul Wilding. The Department allowed us to use its facilities as a base during our most intensive phase of interviewing in the Manchester area. We appreciate this greatly and thank colleagues there for welcoming us.

In the final stages of preparing this book we were able to benefit from the comments of Graham Allan and David Morgan, both of whom undertook to read the whole manuscript. Their perceptive comments helped us to sharpen up our arguments and we are very grateful to both of them.

Jennifer Mason also wishes to thank Caroline Dryden and Andrew Jones who have both taken a long-term interest in the project. Caroline has always been ready and willing to discuss the arguments and analyses we were developing for the book, and has been most generous with her sisterly support. Andrew has amiably endured the writing of the book at close range and has given much appreciated personal support to Jennifer during the writing process. Also he has read and commented on draft chapters, engaged in numerous discussions of the issues on which the book is based, and in general given feedback and input which have helped to clarify and develop the analysis.

Finally, we would like to thank each other for the stimulating and rewarding experience of working together! We have collaborated with each other in the fullest sense of the word in this research project, and in the analysis and writing developed from it. This product is very much a joint one, for which we jointly accept full responsibility.

1 Understanding family responsibilities

INTRODUCTION: WHY STUDY FAMILY RESPONSIBILITIES?

This book is about relationships between members of families in adult life – parents and children, brothers and sisters, aunts, nieces, cousins, grandparents, anyone who is acknowledged as a relative. It is based upon a research study which we have conducted into contemporary relationships between adult kin, especially their significance as sources of practical and financial help. At a time when public statements about the decline in family life are commonplace, we were trying to find out whether these relationships within kin groups do have any real meaning. We were especially interested in whether concepts of family responsibility, or duty or obligation make any sense to people living in contemporary Britain.

To introduce readers to the kind of issues with which the book is concerned, and to illustrate that this is a topic which raises many interesting questions, we begin by giving four brief examples from the data which we have collected. These are not necessarily typical cases or common experiences – indeed each one has some features which are rather unusual. But they are all real. They were stories told to us by people in the late 1980s, to illustrate how structures of practical and financial support worked in their own families. All names are pseudonyms (see Appendix A for details).

Example 1: Sarah Yates and her cousin Mary Mycock

Sarah Yates and Mary Mycock were two cousins, both of whom we interviewed. They were about the same age (in their forties) and both lived with husbands of a second marriage. Each had two children, though Sarah's were older than Mary's and one had already left the parental home. Their homes were about 20 miles apart but both had access to a car. Sarah worked full-time as an ambulance driver. Mary was not doing paid work at the time we interviewed her, and saw looking after her two young children as her full-time job for the moment.

Both of them spoke in warm terms about their relationship over the years. Their contact was not necessarily frequent, but each did always feel that she could call on the other if she needed help. It was a relationship in which various types of assistance had passed in both directions. Mary had made clothes for Sarah's children when they were small, and had agreed to make her elder daughter's wedding dress. They had each looked after the other's children at various different times. Mary used Sarah as her main 'shoulder to cry on' when her first husband left her with little warning. Over the years they had given each other various types of practical, domestic assistance. Sarah gave us a direct illustration of this, when we asked her to tell us what sort of things she and Mary tended to do for each other. She told us that she had just contacted Mary to say that she needed some urgent assistance. She put it this way:

> *Sarah* Well I could tell you what I am doing tonight for instance. My husband has been out there and taken all the plums off the plum tree. And in my garage there's fifty-odd pounds of plums. I'm tied up with this fund-raising I told you about, and all those plums are going to go bad if something's not done with them fast. So I phoned Mary up last night and I said 'If I bring you about forty pounds of plums and the sugar, will you make the jam?' [laughs]. And she said 'Yes' [laughs]. So that's what I'm going up there for tonight [pause]. So that's the sort of thing I mean. We just – just natural, normal, everyday things.

Example 2: Maureen Vickers and her mother

Maureen Vickers was in her early sixties when we interviewed her. She worked full-time for a group of doctors as the administrator of their general practice, and lived in a flat with her unmarried son, who was in his thirties.

Maureen told us in some detail about what had happened when her own mother was terminally ill, many years previously. At that time Maureen was living in London and had a full-time job. Her mother lived in Barrow-in-Furness, more than 300 miles away and in a very inaccessible part of Britain. Maureen had tried to persuade her mother to come and live with her, when she realised that she could no longer cope on her own, but her mother refused. So for two years Maureen and her sister (who also lived near London) managed to look after their mother by an ingenious yet extremely demanding arrangement. Maureen described it like this:

> *Maureen* She had two years in her own home, with her bed downstairs, and I used to go up and look after her for five days. When I left my sister

used to come up. You see, we did it turnabout.

Interviewer Did you actually go and stay at her house?

Maureen At her house yes. I stayed there for five days. And then my sister came and she did her five days [pause]. So that we wouldn't get absolutely bogged down [pause]. Sometimes we used to meet, because there was no train so we had to get the bus, sometimes we used to meet at Levens Bridge. She was getting off one bus and I was waiting for the other. We used to say 'Hi, is she alright?' 'She's fine' [pause]. And this used to be about eleven o'clock at night. On this dark country lane, you know, there could be only one person waiting there. I mean if it wasn't my sister, somebody must have thought 'That's a funny woman over there'.

Example 3: Leona Smith and her brothers

Leona Smith was a young woman in her early twenties, studying for a degree at a college in the north west of England. She had been brought up in Leeds and came from a family of Caribbean descent. Her parents had both migrated to the UK before Leona was born. They had been divorced for some years by the time we interviewed Leona. She had always lived with her mother but also had regular contact with her father.

Leona was the only daughter in this family and had four brothers, three older than herself and one younger. The youngest one was still at school but the older three all had paid jobs – as a cabinet maker, a computer programmer and an electrician. Leona told us how these three brothers, as well as her mother, had all helped her financially during her time at college.

Leona My mum and my brothers, those who have been in employment, have played a major supporting role as regards my education. I do have a grant from the local authority but it is inadequate to deal with everything I require in producing and performing well as a student. Money has been coming regularly from my mum even though I don't ask for it. I think she understands that, as a student you need to do certain things, you need to buy certain books, so she's actually supported me there. So have my brothers – not just financially but they come and see how I am, see if I need anything [pause].

Interviewer The financial help which you get from your brothers, does that come direct to you or is it sort of channelled through your mother?

Leona Oh it's direct to me. Sent in a letter. Sometimes they'll make up the amount my mum sends me in a letter that she writes to me – which is really good.

Example 4: Alf Smith and his mother-in-law

Our last example concerns Alf Smith's relationship with his mother-in-law. He is no relation to Leona Smith. Alf was in his forties when we interviewed him and was living with his wife and his two teenage daughters. He was employed full-time as a gardener for the local council. He had done various manual jobs in the course of his working life, one of which had been as a driver working for a transport company.

Alf told us of an incident which had happened at that time, when he got caught trying to steal a large carton full of packets of butter. He did this while he was picking up a delivery from a warehouse storing grocery products. He planned to sell the butter to the nearest transport cafe, to earn a bit of money on the side. With hindsight Alf considered that he had been stupid to try to steal the butter because he knew that this firm had good security. As a consequence of being caught, he lost his job and was prosecuted for the theft. The court fined him but he had no money to pay. At this point his mother-in-law stepped in to help. Alf told the story like this:

> *Alf*   [After I had been caught] I phoned my firm up and they said 'You're fired'. I said 'Fair comment'. Anyway I finished up in court and it were a fine of five pounds, which I hadn't got at the time. Two days to pay. I thought 'Where am I going to get five pounds in two days?' No job, sort of thing. Well down at my mother-in-law's, it were the wife, she called at her mother's coming home [pause] and she were telling her all this. My mother-in-law, straight into her purse, you know. She said 'There you are. Tell that lad to get straight up to the courts and pay his fine. And he can pay me the money when he's got it.'

These four stories are in many ways very different. They concern different relationships – parents and children, brothers and sisters, in-laws, cousins. They are about very different types of help – money, practical assistance, looking after someone who is ill. The circumstances outlined are very diverse – from 'natural, normal, everyday things' (as Sarah Yates puts it) to a case where the need is extreme, like the care of a dying elderly woman. What they have in common is that they are all examples of one relative helping another. At the very least, they show that in these four families, kin relationships do have some significance in adult life as the means through which people receive various types of assistance.

But examples like these raise issues beyond the simple observation that, at least for some people and in some situations, kin relationships can 'work' as support mechanisms. We can see this by posing the more analytical question: what is going on here? This can be developed in several ways. We can ask for example: in what sense are any or all of these people helping their relatives *because* they are relatives? We might imagine that Maureen Vickers is unlikely to take on the kind of caring role which she decribes for someone who is not a relative; possibly she would not do it for anyone other than a parent. This reasoning also may apply to other examples – the fact that people are related seems central to understanding why they help each other. But what about Sarah Yates and Mary Mycock? Is the fact that they are cousins of any real importance in understanding the nature of their relationship and the assistance which they give to each other? Or are we really looking at a pattern of mutual aid which could just as easily grow up between two friends? They happen to be cousins, but this may be of little relevance to understanding what is going on between them.

Even in those examples where we might feel more confident about saying that help is given *because* the person in need is a relative, can we assume that the help flows from a sense of family duty or responsibility? Are the people who provide help doing it because they feel that they 'ought to', that they have an obligation to help a relative which would not apply to other people? Again in a case like Maureen Vickers' the idea that her actions flow from a sense of duty seems quite plausible. It seems much less plausible to see Alf Smith's mother-in-law in that light. Does she really pay off Alf's fine because she feels a sense of duty to the son-in-law to whom she refers as 'that lad'? Or is she actually more concerned about the reputation of her family in the eyes of her friends and neighbours, and therefore keen to see that the fine does get paid? Or perhaps her real concern is to ensure that there is not too much financial pressure on the household where her grandchildren are being brought up. If a sense of duty is involved here, it may be a sense of duty to her daughter and her grand-daughters rather than to her son-in-law, who is the person she actually helps.

Translated into more general terms, these are the kind of questions with which we began the research whose findings we discuss in this book. They were questions which we were interested in before we heard any of the stories which we have told here. Our interest in pursuing them stemmed from intellectual questions which have their foundations in sociological writings and in the analysis of social policy. We will now spell out these intellectual underpinnings of our work, and address the question 'why study family responsibilities?' in a more formal way.

We begin by clarifying what we mean by the term 'family' in this context. We are focusing on relationships in adult life, so our work is not about responsibilities for young children. Also we have not been concerned specifically to study the responsibilities of spouses, though clearly these cannot be totally excluded if one is interested (which we are) in the overall pattern of responsibilities which develop in a family. Strictly, therefore, our work is about kinship. If we were being precise we would use only the word 'kin' throughout this book. However we have chosen to use it interchangeably with 'family' and 'relatives' because these are the words most commonly in use among the general population to describe the relationships which we are studying. None of the people we interviewed actually used the term kin. They did use 'family' and 'relatives' extensively – sometimes interchangeably, sometimes drawing a distinction between 'family' who are close and 'relatives' who are more distant (Firth, Hubert and Forge, 1970).

We wanted to concentrate principally on responsibilities associated with adult relationships with relatives for three main reasons. First, much less is known about them than about relationships associated with the nuclear family household. A number of well-known studies of family, kinship and community were conducted in the 1950s and 1960s (Young and Willmott, 1957; Stacey, 1960; Bell, 1968; Rosser and Harris, 1968; Firth, Hubert and Forge, 1970) but then this type of research fell out of fashion. Most research concerned with family relationships in recent years has concentrated on the household, thus necessarily focusing mainly on spouses and on parents with young children (for good summaries of this work, see Brannen and Wilson, 1987; Morris, 1990).

Our second reason for screening out parents' responsibilities for young children, and responsibilities between spouses, was that these relationships have a special status in that the responsibilities which they entail are subject to legal definition. The responsibilities attached to other adult kin relationships are not legally defined in Britain, or at least they have not been since 1948 when the Poor Law was formally abolished. Before that there was a legal expectation that, if the need arose, children were responsible for giving their parents financial assistance, and grandparents as well as parents had a responsibility to support children of immature years. In Victorian Britain the Poor Law authorities attempted to enforce these responsibilities in order to ensure that as few people as possible became a charge on public funds (Wall, 1977; Quadagno, 1982). But since 1948, the responsibilities associated with relationships outside the nuclear family and the household have not been systematically defined in law. Yet it is possible to find examples – like those which we used at the beginning of this chapter – which show that they can be channels through which significant forms of assistance pass, and within which people do appear to operate with a concept of family responsibilities.

Our third reason for being interested in relationships between adult kin concerns the type of social and economic changes which have occurred in the period when little social research on kinship has been conducted in Britain. Interesting and important though the earlier generation of studies is, we cannot assume that its findings are relevant to understanding kinship in the 1980s and 1990s. In the intervening thirty years a good deal has happened in British society which may have had some impact on kin relationships – urban development, shifts of population across the country, an economic recession, the rapid growth in the numbers of elderly people, significant shifts in the political climate, the creation of a multi-ethnic society through the migration and settlement of people from Asia, Africa and the Caribbean.

The effects of these changes on kin relationships are not easy to predict. On the one hand we might expect factors such as geographical mobility and the break-up of settled communities through redevelopment, to mean that kin relationships have become more fragmented and of less importance in the last thirty years. The earlier generation of kinship studies certainly picked up on the beginning of such patterns (see especially Willmott and Young, 1960). On the other hand some of the social and economic pressures which we have identified might work in the opposite direction. Economic hardship caused by a recession could perhaps mean that more people have had to rely on their kin for help. The increased numbers of elderly people in the population, at a time when the government has been trying to hold down public expenditure, has meant an explicit shift in social policies, to encourage families to take greater responsibility for the care of their elderly relatives. This shift can be traced through a number of policy proposals and is well documented (see for example, Finch and Groves, 1980; Henwood and Wicks, 1985; Ungerson, 1990). In so far as such policies are successful, one might expect to find that kin relationships have become more, not less, important. The tensions which can be created between contradictory pressures – geographical mobility on the one hand, responsibility for the care of an elderly parent on the other – are illustrated graphically in the case of Maureen Vickers, which we presented earlier.

In searching for research of more recent origin on kin relationships and how they are changing, one finds very little which addresses these issues directly. Contemporary kinship therefore is a topic about which little is known, and one where there is a clear need to update earlier work. Yet the case for studying family responsibilities does not rest solely on the updating argument. Beyond that there is a range of questions about the nature of kin relationships specifically which make them an intellectually interesting and important topic for study. The book *Family Obligations and Social Change*, which Janet Finch wrote while we were conducting our research (Finch, 1989), explores some of these questions in considerable detail as well as reviewing existing evidence about kin relationships and obligations. In a sense that book forms the background to our study and we are not going to offer a discussion of the same literature here. We shall simply refer readers to Finch (1989) where we think appropriate links can be made. Indeed we can go much further here because we have acquired a rich data set which enables us both to examine similar analytical questions to those addressed in Finch (1989), and to pose and address new ones. But also, it is here that we jointly develop our own theoretical position, in the light of our data.

The particular set of intellectual questions with which we engage in this book concern kin responsibilities and how they operate in practice. As we put it in discussing the examples at the beginning of this chapter: where people give help to their relatives, do they do it *because* they are kin, and what are the foundations of such assistance? This links with a key debate in classic social anthropology, about whether kin relationships should be seen as a special category of social relationships, characterised by feelings of obligation and duty which do not apply to other relationships. The obligation which distinctively characterises kinship, it is argued, is an obligation to share resources and to give assistance when it is needed, without thought of personal gain. The view is expressed succinctly by Fortes, one of its major proponents, 'What I wish to stress is the basic premise: kinship is binding; it creates inescapable moral claims and obligations' (Fortes, 1969: 242).

Against this, other anthropologists have argued that kin relationships do not have this distinctive 'moral character' but can be explained in the same way as all others – ultimately they are concerned with the material and economic interests of individuals. (Key sources in this debate are: Worsley, 1956; Leach, 1961; Fortes, 1969; Bloch, 1973).

The idea that kin relationships do have a distinctive character which marks them off from all others, and that this character is defined in terms of moral rules concerned with duty and obligation, finds echoes in many other places. It certainly has underscored the thinking of politicians and policy-makers, as they have sought to draw a line between the responsibilities which the state is going to assume for the welfare of its citizens, and those which can be presumed to be taken care of by the family. We have already referred to the Victorian Poor Law as an example of kin responsibilities being enshrined in the law. It can be shown that lying behind this was a belief that an intrinsic part of being a husband, or a daughter, or a father, is that one recognises an obligation to give assistance when it is needed (Finch, 1989). It is the concept of the moral character of kinship translated into social policy and the law.

The abolition of the Poor Law has not completely removed such thinking. Indeed many people have argued – though they have put it in different language – that this principle has been strongly reasserting itself as governments in Britain and in many other Western countries have sought to re-draw the line between state responsibilities and family responsibilities, and to encourage people to see the family as the first line of assistance on which they should call, both practically and financially. This can apply in a number of different circumstances, but most obviously the pressure in social policy has come first, in relation to the care of the growing number of infirm elderly people, and second, in respect of providing housing and economic assistance for young adults who cannot yet fully support themselves (see for example, Morgan, 1985; Wallace, 1987; Harris, 1988; Finch, 1990). In both these situations it is being assumed that the strength of family ties, and the sense of responsibility which they incorporate, will be sufficient in most cases to ensure that people's needs are met. In the eyes of some politicans at least, the case for doing so is bolstered by an ideological commitment to strengthening family life which – some people argue – is being eroded because people have been able to rely too much on the state (Parker, 1986; Anderson, 1990). It is not too difficult to see that the potential implications of this are very different for women and for men.

This view of family responsibilities – as rules of contact associated with genealogical relationships – in many ways seems very crude, though it is important because it has been so influential. However it is possible to draw on other types of social theory and develop a concept of responsibility and obligation which has somewhat different features. Janet Finch explored this in her book on *Family Obligations and Social Change* (1989:142–78). She argued that existing research suggests that in practice people operate with a concept of family obligation which is much more fluid than is implied by the ideas of moral rules associated with genealogical positions. The concept of 'guidelines' is more appropriate than rules, she suggested. The available evidence suggested that it is not possible to identify clear rules about *what* someone should do for a relative in defined circumstances. But people do seem to acknowledge guidelines, in the sense of considerations which it is appropriate to take into account in working out whether to offer assistance to a relative.

Thus the case for researching family responsibilities has both an intellectual and a policy dimension. Intellectually there are some interesting and important questions about whether kin relationships do have a distinctive character, and if so, what is special about them. These are questions about whether kin relationships are distinctively defined in terms of obligations and responsibilities; if so, to whom these apply, and in what circumstances; and whether concepts like 'following rules' or 'using guidelines' make any sense of how people relate to kin in practice. In posing questions in this form, we are implying different possible meanings for concepts like obligation and responsibility, and we explore these in subsequent chapters. These intellectual questions imply that we need to know what family responsibilities people acknowledge in principle and what are their practical consequences. The answers to such questions are also important in policy terms in a situation where governments seek to place more weight upon family responsibilities. It is quite possible that assumptions are being made, and incorporated into social policies, which do not align with the ways in which kin relationships operate in practice, and which contain unrealistic expectations about what kin will do for each other. In policy terms it is important to know whether this is happening in the 1980s and 1990s. It is not enough simply to assume that the family as a social institution is ready, willing and able to shoulder the burden of supporting its members who cannot fully care for themselves, either practically or financially.

These issues about family responsibilities can only be addressed adequately on the basis of empirical evidence. Our own research tried to address them by posing empirical questions such as the following. In the context of the late twentieth century in Britain, what responsibilities *are* most of us prepared to acknowledge towards our relatives? Do we think that relatives have a right to make claims upon us, or we on them? Which relatives? What sort of claims? How does all this work out in practice? Does the whole concept of 'family responsibilities' have any meaning or significance in most of our lives? Should any of these questions be answered differently for women and men? We designed a piece of research which, we believed, would enable us to provide some answers to them. We are using the rest of this chapter to introduce our research and to present some key findings in a preliminary way.

THE FAMILY OBLIGATIONS PROJECT

The research on which this book is based was known as the Family Obligations Project. We were collecting data for this study between 1985 and 1988 and our fieldwork was located in the geographical area defined as Greater Manchester. This is a region in the north west of England with nearly three million inhabitants. It covers the cities of Manchester and Salford, a ring of small towns round it (Bolton, Bury, Oldham, Rochdale, Stockport) and the rural areas between them. A few interviews were conducted in Preston, a town marginally outside this region. The region was the centre of the cotton industry in the earlier industrial period and the towns mentioned experienced the urban growth associated with the industrial revolution from the early nineteenth century. More details of the location, and of the design of our study as a whole, are given in Appendix A. The study was located in Greater Manchester only, but this region is reasonably representative of the UK as a whole in terms of social, economic and ethnic composition, and the questions which we are tackling are big ones, raising issues which are important nationally and internationally.

The design of our project reflected the research questions which we were posing, and which we have set out in the previous section, about giving and receiving help in kin groups. We included help of all kinds: giving and lending money, occasional or regular help with domestic tasks and child care, offering a home temporarily or permanently to a relative who has nowhere to live, giving personal care to someone who cannot look after themselves. We wanted to include a wide range of circumstances in adult life where such assistance might be given – between different generations and between people in the same generation.

Our study was in two main parts, a large-scale survey and an in-depth qualitative study. We will describe each of them very briefly here, but more details are given in Appendix A. The purpose of the two halves of the study was very different, and together they give us a rich data set. In the survey we were aiming to find out whether, in Britain of the 1980s, we could identify any kind of consensus about family obligations and responsibilities. Do people have a clear sense about what constitute appropriate responsibilities and obligations towards relatives? Is there any kind of agreement about 'the proper thing to do', when faced with a relative who has a particular need? We thought it important to pose these questions because assumptions were being made in social policy which imply that there is indeed a consensus over these matters.

This type of research question, focused on the issue of whether there is consensus or agreement about principles of family responsibilities, implied that we needed to study a representative sample of the general population, hence the decision to pursue these questions through a large-scale survey. This was based on a sample from the electoral register in forty wards in Greater Manchester, and therefore included a cross-section of people from the age of 18 upwards. In total we interviewed 978 people, a respectable response rate of 72 per cent. On most criteria, our survey population was a reasonable reflection of the general population (see Appendix A for some details of the comparison), although of course it is not necessarily representative of sub-groups within that population.

The research issues which we were trying to address through the survey were about the norms and beliefs to which people give public assent. We were *not* trying to use the survey to find out details about people's relationships with their own kin, nor even about how people incorporate normative beliefs into their own family relationships. The type of questions which we asked reflected this aim. Most of the questions in these interviews were based on some version of the vignette technique (Finch, 1987a), where we presented our respondents with a situation where someone is in need of practical or financial help. We then posed questions which invited them to consider matters such as: should relatives provide help in these kinds of circumstances? which relatives? what should they do and why? A simple example would be this question:

Suppose that a young couple with a small child have returned from working abroad and can't afford to buy or rent anywhere to live until one of them gets a job. Should any of their relatives offer to have the family in their home for the next few months?

If respondents answered 'yes' to this, we then went on to ask them which relatives should be the first to offer help.

In posing this type of question, we hoped to be able to determine whether there is agreement about 'the proper thing to do' in a given set of circumstances. We used hypothetical questions about third parties and asked people to respond by telling us *what these people should do*. We did not want to ask what our respondents themselves *would* do because the answers of each would inevitably be coloured by his or her own family circumstances and tied to their own experience. In posing hypothetical questions about third parties, we were trying to elicit data on whether there is agreement that *if* a given set of circumstances arises, there is an obvious and proper way of responding. That is what we mean when we say that we were trying to use the survey to tap publicly expressed norms about family responsibilities.

Though we focused upon publicly expressed norms in the survey, we saw this as only part of the picture at which we wanted to look. This type of research can tap beliefs at one level – the level at which people acknowledge publicly what is right and proper for third parties. But it does not tell us whether or how such beliefs get translated into relationships within families, or how far they are reflected in the responsibilities which people acknowledge for their own relatives. Hence the other part of our study, which was designed to understand how people develop commitments and responsibilities towards their relatives in practice. In developing a framework for studying this dimension, we focused on the idea that kin responsibilities have negotiated as well as normative elements. We based this idea, for example, on findings from the earlier generation of kinship studies, in particular that of Firth, Hubert and Forge (1970), where the authors concluded that kin relationships in Britain tend to be 'permissive not obligatory'. By this they meant that there is an absence of clear rules about precisely who should do what for whom. In the absence of such rules, we reasoned, it follows that people have to *work out* what type of responsibilities they are going to acknowledge to particular relatives. Family responsibilities thus become a matter for negotiation between individuals and not just a matter of following normative rules (for further elaboration of these arguments see Finch, 1987b, 1989: 179–211).

Thus a central theme of the second part of our study was to explore the proposition that such commitments are the result of processes of negotiation in families. Given that our aim was to study *processes* within families in this part of the research, we had to take an approach very different from the survey. Surveys offer an important means of studying certain types of research question, but it is well recognised that they are ill-suited to uncovering the dynamics of social processes. We therefore developed a study which relied on qualitative research methods, principally using semi-structured interviewing techniques.

Our qualitative study includes eighty-eight people, some of them interviewed more than once. We conducted the interviews ourselves. In contrast with the survey, at this stage of the research we were making no attempt to construct a study population which would be representative in a statistical sense. Our procedure for selecting interviewees was complex, and is discussed in more detail in Appendix A and also in Finch and Mason (1990a). We selected initially from people who had been in the survey then, having re-interviewed them once, in some cases we asked permission to approach their relatives with a view to interviewing them as well. The relatives whom we approached were usually those whom our initial contact person had identified as her or his close family. Thus, of the eighty-eight people in this part of the study, some are there as individuals and others have relatives included in the study. In total we included eleven 'kin groups' where we interviewed between three and eight members of the same family. We believed that there would be great benefit in interviewing several members of the same family, since we were focusing upon processes of negotiation and therefore we needed to know how these were experienced by different parties to them. Much previous work on family relationships has been criticised because researchers have interviewed just one person from each family – usually a woman – and just let that person's account stand for the whole family group. We were anxious to avoid that in our own work.

Appendix A gives details of how we selected interviewees initially and how we arrived at the eleven 'kin groups'. But we would like to underline here what we mean by a 'kin group' in the context of our study. Essentially it is *one person's* kin group, the person who was our initial point of contact. We invited that person to define whom she or he 'counted' as their family, and took that as our definition of the group we were interested in studying. If we had begun with a different person within that group, we almost certainly would have got a slightly different definition of who counted as their kin. Thus when we refer to one of our 'kin groups' we do not mean to imply that it has any existence as 'a group' other than in the context of our research. But the relationships within it most certainly do have an independent reality.

The content of our interviews with the people in the qualitative study focused principally upon their own families, though we did also repeat one or two questions which had been in the survey. For most of the interview, we simply asked people to tell us about relationships in their own families, concentrating upon examples of support and assistance which they and others had experienced. We tried then to draw them out on questions concerning their own sense of responsibility to relatives and how this had been arrived at. (More details are given in Appendix A.) These interviews were tape-recorded and fully transcribed and we have already quoted from some of them in the four examples which we gave at the beginning of this chapter.

The two parts of the study were designed as a complementary whole, enabling us to look at both public and private meanings of 'family', to compare expressed beliefs with the realities of relationships in practice, to understand both the normative and the negotiated elements of family responsibilities. We were particularly concerned to keep a clear distinction between beliefs and actions and not to make the common mistake of assuming that actions can be 'read off' from beliefs. We were clear that the kind of beliefs about family responsibilities which people express in a survey cannot be used to predict what they themselves do in their own lives. The foundations of social action are much more complex than that. Yet there may well be *some* relationship between the two. The design of our study makes it possible to explore issues such as that.

In presenting our findings, we have tried to capitalise on the complementary character of our data set by discussing the survey data and the interview data side by side. We do this in different ways in different chapters. For the rest of this first chapter we introduce the findings from both halves of our study, and provide an illustration of the potential of this data set for answering the kind of questions which we have posed. We begin with some key findings from the survey data.

PUBLIC NORMS AND FAMILY RESPONSIBILITIES

Is there a clear consensus among the British population about what kind of responsibilities people should acknowledge towards their relatives? Our survey was designed centrally to address this issue and – briefly but firmly – the answer is no. In answers given by a representative sample of the adult population, there are remarkably few circumstances in which people are in agreement that the responsibility to give help lies clearly with relatives. We have discussed aspects of our survey data in articles in journals, and we will draw on these in summarising the main features here. Readers who want more specific detail might care to consult those articles (Finch and Mason, 1990b, 1990c, 1990d, 1991).

We can demonstrate that there is a lack of consensus about family responsibilities by looking first simply at the proportion of questions where there was a high level of agreement among our survey respondents. In total our survey contained sixty-nine questions, or parts of questions, which focused on normative issues. The answers to 48 per cent of these show no consensus. In the remaining 52 per cent where there is some agreement, when we look at *what* people are saying about family responsibilities, no clear patterns emerge. Answers do not point consistently in the same direction and messages are mixed.

At this point we should say what we mean by 'consensus' or a 'high level of agreement'. In asking questions about family responsibilities we are very unlikely to find 100 per cent consensus. So how many people have to agree with each other before we will count it as a high level of agreement – 90 per cent? 75 per cent? 50 per cent? This is not straightforwardly a statistical question. It is more a matter of how data are interpreted.

We have developed a rule of thumb for interpretation using the idea of a 'consensus baseline' (Finch and Mason, 1991). Briefly, we have reasoned that where we posed a question just inviting a yes/no answer (or in any other way gave respondents only two options), anything more than 50 per cent saying either 'yes' or 'no' would represent a simple majority. However, a split of something like 52 per cent against 48 per cent could hardly be regarded as a high level of agreement in either direction. Thus we need something substantially more than 50 per cent, but less than 100 per cent, to say that we would 'count' it as a high level of agreement. We decided to use the principle that, where an answer attracts at least one-and-a-half times the simple majority, we will take this as indicating significant agreement. In the case of two-option questions, this gives us a figure of 75 per cent as our consensus baseline. Where we were giving respondents the choice of three different answers, the corresponding figure is 50 per cent, and for four-option questions it is 37.5 per cent. We have proceeded with our analysis using these 'consensus baseline' figures, but we must emphasise that we see them as a starting-point for interpretation, and an aid to it, not as the ultimate arbiter of what agreement means.

As we have indicated, of a possible sixty-nine survey questions, 48 per cent had a pattern of answers which reached our consensus baseline and 52 per cent did not. In this section we are not attempting an overview of all sixty-nine questions but will concentrate on a group of fourteen, which are the key questions for our purpose here. Details of these questions, and the answers to them, are given in Appendix B. All of these are short questions (as opposed to our more complex questions and longer vignettes) where we sketched out a situation where someone needs financial or practical help, and then asked respondents to say *whether* it should come from relatives. Sometimes we simply asked whether relatives should help or not; sometimes we suggested a specific alternative source such as borrowing money from a bank, or state-provided support services for an infirm person. Thus these questions help us to focus directly on the issue of whether people see relatives as the appropriate way of providing assistance *rather than* the use of some other source.

In these fourteen questions some answers reached our consensus baseline and others did not. We will give some examples of the range of answers given to these questions, beginning with the two in which there was clear agreement that relatives *should* be the people to provide help. The highest level of agreement was in the question, which we quoted earlier in this chapter, about a young couple returning from abroad and having nowhere to live: 86 per cent of our respondents said that relatives should offer a temporary home (consensus baseline 75 per cent). The other question in which there was agreement that relatives should help concerned a 19-year-old girl with a baby. We said that she had been living with her boyfriend but the relationship had broken up, leaving her without a home and without money. We asked whether she should go to her parents' home or do something else; 79 per cent said that she should go back to her parents' home. We then asked those people who said that she should do something else whether her parents should offer a home, and 77 per cent of them said that they should (consensus baseline 75 per cent on both parts of this question). Thus there were high levels of agreement among our survey population that the parents should make their home available to their daughter, even among people who actually thought that the daughter should not accept this offer.

The fact that there are only two questions – out of a possible fourteen – where our respondents clearly preferred the idea of assistance from relatives to other alternatives indicates that there is no real consensus that the family should normally be the first line of support for people in need. At the same time our survey respondents were not straightforwardly rejecting the idea of family responsibilities. Out of the fourteen questions which we are considering here, only two produced a clear agreement that relatives are *not* the appropriate source of help (see Appendix B).

The majority of the questions – ten in all – in fact show what we are calling a 'split consensus', that is a pattern of answers in which views vary about whether relatives are the most appropriate source of help. Often people were split quite evenly on the question of whether relatives should step in and offer assistance in defined circumstances. For example, one question read like this:

> If an elderly person, who has become very frail, and can only move around with help, can no longer live alone should she or he move into an old people's home or go and live with relatives?

Only 27 per cent said that this elderly person should live with relatives, and twice as many (55 per cent) said that she or he should move into an old people's home. But neither of these figures reaches our consensus baseline of 75 per cent and as many as 10 per cent were uncertain, or said that it would depend on circumstances. Thus our survey population was very divided on the appropriate source of help in these cirumstances. Where respondents had chosen 'old people's home' we asked whether there are any circumstances under which this elderly person should live with relatives. Their answers were split just about equally between yes and no, further reinforcing the impression that there is no clear agreement about the role of relatives in providing help in these circumstances. Similar split consensus patterns are found in the other ten questions in this group, some of which are about accommodation as this question was, some about practical and personal support, and some about financial assistance. Details can be found in Appendix B.

Thus the clear impression from our data is that norms and beliefs about family responsibilities are not easily recognised or clearly agreed upon among the British population. However, it is possible that the kind of patterns which we found could be related to the characteristics of our respondents in a systematic way. The common pattern of split consensus suggests that our data may be reflecting two or three different sets of normative ideas among our survey respondents. For example, do women and men answer these questions differently? Is there a split in beliefs about family responsibilities along social class lines? Do people who themselves have received considerable help from their families think differently from others about the issue of responsibilities and obligations?

We did gather information about our respondents which would help us to consider these questions, but it shows that there are no very clear patterns. Somewhat to our surprise, gender seems to be of little importance at this level of tapping the kind of norms which people express in response to survey questions. On some questions there are some variations in the pattern of men's and women's answers – usually quite small – but in other cases there is little difference. However, when we put together the answers where there *is* variation, no consistent messages emerge. We know from many other sources that, in practice, women are more likely to give relatives practical and personal support than are men (Green, 1988; Arber and Gilbert, 1989). However, it seems from our survey that the explanation of this does not lie at the level of publicly acknowledged norms. Women and men apparently endorse similar beliefs and values at this level. Thus we need to look elsewhere for explanations of the differences observed in practice. Similarly there is little systematic difference in answers given by people with different social class backgrounds, defined in conventional terms. (See Finch and Mason, 1991 for more detailed discussion of this issue.)

On the question of people's own experience, and whether that affects the views which they express in a survey about family responsibilities, it is obviously difficult to know precisely what kind of experiences might be relevant, and whether we have collected enough information about each respondent to pick these up. We did ask some limited questions about people's own experience of family life – about whether they had given or received assistance in the form of money, accommodation or personal care. We are rather cautious about using these as they flatten out what may be very disparate types of experience, and it could well be that some of our respondents who did not report such experiences had in fact had them – survey methods in general are not well suited to collecting this type of information. But so far as we can tell from what was reported to us, the experience of giving or receiving assistance with accommodation or personal care has little effect on the way people answered our questions about family responsibilities. In questions about money, there does seem to be some relationship. Where respondents themselves had given or lent a fairly substantial sum of money to a relative (we specified £300 or more) they were more likely than other people to favour relatives giving financial assistance in our questions about hypothetical situations (Finch and Mason, 1991).

In general, therefore, the rather mixed and apparently contradictory pattern of answers in our survey is not explained by different groups of respondents giving different answers. What seems to be happening is that people were making judgements about the appropriateness of family assistance in the light of the circumstances which we outlined in each question. There are *some circumstances* in which most people do agree that the family should take responsibility, as for example the case of the young couple returning from abroad and needing a temporary home. But there is no evidence at all of a general feeling that the family should normally be the first port of call for most people.

We need to look therefore at those circumstances in which people do tend to agree that the family should be the first line of assistance. Do they have any common features? Looking across the whole range of our survey data, three interesting features stand out. First, it seems most likely that people will endorse family responsibilities in 'deserving cases' where the need is presented as entirely legitimate and the person who needs assistance is not at fault in any way. Our young family returning from overseas meets these criteria very clearly. Their situation contrasts with that of another hypothetical young family who, we said, needed money to pay for a long-awaited holiday. In this case we had a high level of agreement that they should 'do without the holiday' rather than seek financial assistance from relatives. We see this as indicating that a holiday was seen as a luxury item rather than a clear and legitimate need. We can also draw a contrast with another question concerning a family with young children who needed a temporary home because they had been evicted for non-payment of rent. In this case 65 per cent said that relatives should offer help – a figure which did not reach our consensus baseline and contrasts with the 86 per cent who said that relatives should offer a home to the young couple returning from overseas. We would argue that the difference between these two figures reflects a feeling on the part of some respondents that the family evicted from their home were less deserving because they were somewhat responsible for their own circumstances.

The second feature which emerges from our data is that people are more likely to accord responsibility to relatives when the assistance needed is fairly limited – in terms of time, effort or skill. In the question about the young couple returning from abroad we specified that they needed a home 'for a few months'. In other questions it was less clear that, for example, an offer to give someone accommodation would be time-limited. In questions about caring for someone who cannot fully look after themselves, our respondents were more likely to accord responsibility to relatives if the assistance needed was temporary, or did not demand high levels of skill. But in questions which implied that the person needed *nursing* care, including intimate bodily contact, more people were inclined to say that state services were preferable to relatives.

Third, our data do support the view that responsibilities between parents and children are accorded a special status. This is in line with earlier research on kinship which indicates that, although in general relationships are permissive not obligatory, parent–child relationships come closest to having fixed responsibilities associated with them (Morgan, 1975). In questions where we asked people to identify *which* relatives should provide assitance in adult life, parents or children were much more likely to be named than any other (Finch and Mason, 1990b, 1991).

However, in our data it is clear that people do not see parent–child responsibilities as automatic or unlimited. We put the the following proposition to our respondents and asked them to agree or disagree on a five-point scale:

Children have no obligation to look after their parents when they are old.

The response to this was one of our 'split consensus' items: 58 per cent of our respondents said that children *do* have an obligation to look after their parents but 39 per cent said that they *do not*. In other questions about children looking after elderly parents, people tended to agree that children had a responsibility to do *something*, but views varied on *what* they should do. For example in one question (which we discuss in detail in Chapter 3), we posed a dilemma of whether a son and his wife should take any responsibility for his parents, who had both been injured in a car accident and lived several hundred miles away. Most of our respondents favoured an option in which they did take some responsibility – only 9 per cent said that they should 'let the parents make their own arrangements'. But as to precisely what they should do, our respondents were evenly divided between the other three options which we offered: move to live near the husband's parents 33 per cent; have the parents move to live with them 24 per cent; give the parents money to help them pay for their daily care 25 per cent.

There is some evidence in our survey data that we should not treat parent–child relationships as symmetrical in terms of responsibilities. The two examples in Appendix B where there is agreement that relatives *should* help concern parents helping a child in young adult life – the young couple returning from abroad and needing a temporary home, and the young woman with a baby who also needs a home. In one of our longer vignettes (which we discuss in detail in Chapter 5) we posed a situation about a man called John Highfield who was in his early thirties and needed financial help to start his own business. This question attracted high levels of agreement that his parents were appropriate people to lend him money. By contrast we have split patterns of responses in all the questions in Appendix B which pose the issue of whether older people should seek help from their children rather than elsewhere.

Thus there is a sense in which, at this level of publicly acknowledged norms about family life, parents' continuing responsibility to help their children seems to be endorsed more strongly and more predictably than any other type of family responsibility. However, even here there are clear limits especially, it would seem, to do with 'deservingness' or 'genuine need'. The question about a young student getting into debt (see Appendix B) led to a mixed pattern of responses with 65 per cent saying that his parents should *not* pay off the debts (consensus baseline 75 per cent). Further, the two questions in Appendix B which attracted a high level of agreement that relatives should *not* help concerned couples in young adult life, one wanting money to pay for a holiday, the other to pay private school fees. We have to be careful about interpretation here, since in these questions we asked whether 'relatives' should help and did not specify parents. Nonetheless we know from other questions that parents would be seen as the most likely source of help in such circumstances. In both instances, the message was firmly that these are not cases of 'genuine need' and therefore that relatives have no obligation to help: 67 per cent of our respondents said that the first couple should do without the holiday and 79 per cent said that the second couple should keep their children in state schools.

In summary, in responding to these survey questions a representative sample of the population was telling us that, even when it comes to parent–child responsibilities, there are no clear rules about what you should do. At this point it is useful to refer to the distinction between rules which tell you *what* you should do and guidelines which indicate *how to work out* the proper thing to do in a given set of circumstances. In analysing our survey data, we are referring to the former as substantive issues and the latter as procedural issues, and we believe that our data show higher levels of agreement on procedural than on substantive matters (Finch and Mason, 1991). The first two significant features of our data which we outlined above – deserving cases and commitments being limited – can be expressed as procedural guidelines. We can turn them round and say that, when faced with a decision about whether a relative should feel an obligation to offer help most people think that it is appropriate to consider matters such as: is this a case of legitimate need? is it a luxury or a necessity? is this person in need of assistance through no fault of their own? how big a commitment would an offer of help entail? If the person in need is a parent or a child, the test to be passed may be less stringent but on the whole it is still appropriate to ask this kind of question.

Thus we can say with some confidence that our survey data show that there is nothing approaching a clear consensus about family responsibilities. In the late 1980s in Britain people apparently were not acknowledging clearly identifiable principles about what kinds of assistance family members should offer each other. There is no evidence of a clear acknowledgement at this public normative level that families should be the first line of support for their members. This is something of a contrast with assumptions made in social policy. Leaving aside the question of what people will actually be prepared to do in practice it seems that, even at this level, relatives cannot be relied upon to acknowledge that they have clear responsibilities.

FAMILY RESPONSIBILITIES IN PRACTICE: A CASE EXAMPLE

As we have explained, our study was set up on the assumption that understanding family responsibilities requires us to look at different dimensions, using different kinds of data. Our survey gives us important data about publicly expressed norms, which help us to answer key questions about family responsibilities especially as they relate to questions of public policy. But these kind of data can tell us very little about how commitments and responsibilities develop in practice. As we have indicated, we see processes of negotiation in families as central to understanding this, and this view is supported by some of the messages coming out of our survey data.

The message that 'circumstances' are highly relevant to determining which responsibilities relatives should acknowledge points to the importance of looking at negotiations within families. So too does our observation that there is more agreement over procedures than over the substance of obligations.

Our qualitative study was designed to enable us to look at family responsibilities in this way. To conclude this chapter we are going to present a preliminary example from our qualitative data set. We are using this as a way of illustrating the kind of questions which can be addressed with data of this type, and as a means of demonstrating how our two data sets mesh together and enable us to answer complex questions about family responsibilities. In the course of doing this inevitably we throw up questions which we cannot deal with fully in this preliminary example, but which point the way to some themes taken up in later chapters.

Our example comes from the Gardner kin group, where we interviewed Tim, who was in his early twenties, and his parents, Lawrence and Caroline. Tim was their only child. Though of course all families have unique features, there was nothing strikingly unusual about this family. Certainly they saw themselves as very ordinary. Tim had graduated from university about eighteen months previously and, at the time we interviewed him, was running a small business on an Enterprise Allowance. Tim acknowledged that the business was not doing very well. We interviewed him twice and by the time of the second interview, suspecting that the business might not keep going when he could no longer claim the Enterprise Allowance, he was beginning to apply for jobs and anticipating a possible career in management. During his time at university Tim had had one year working full-time as the social secretary of the students' union. He had been brought up in the Greater Manchester region, in the house where his parents still lived. Lawrence was a self-employed upholsterer, having taken on his own father's small business. Caroline was a trained dress-maker, working sometimes for Lawrence, sometimes for other employers, and sometimes had periods when she did not work for wages.

In our discussion here we are concentrating upon Tim's relationship with his parents over questions of money and economic support. Tim was in the process of moving into independent adult life when we did our interviews – a process which was quite protracted in his case because he had had four years at university, followed by a period where he was attempting to establish himself as self-employed. The questions upon which we shall focus are: what responsibility did Tim's parents feel for giving him financial support during this period when he was becoming established as an adult? what responsibilities did they feel for securing his financial future in the longer term? through what means had these commitments been arrived at?

how were they understood by each of the three parties involved? did the responsibilities acknowledged now have any implications for the relationship between Tim and his parents in the future?

All three Gardners told us about their financial relationships, Tim and Caroline both talking about this issue quite extensively. Tim's parents had obviously given him a considerable amount of help and were continuing to do so. While he was a student, though he was entitled to a grant and ultimately he received it, it was not clear that he would get one because the assessment of his parents' income was complex, principally because his father was self-employed. In Tim's view also his father's accountant was 'very incompetent'. Thus he went through most of his student career without being certain whether he was going to receive money from his local authority. Lawrence and Caroline could not afford to support him out of their own resources but felt a strong responsibility to ensure that he was able to take up his university place. So Caroline took a sewing job in a factory to meet Tim's expenses. As she put it herself:

> *Caroline* I had to go back to work because Lawrence could not keep us and pay for him, which is what I did. I went back to work and my entire wages just kept Tim in his hall of residence [pause]. We worked it out and over a year, we knew that the rent was roughly three hundred and something pounds for each term [pause]. And we decided that, three years ago it wasn't so bad, that he could live on between £25 and £30 a week [pause]. So I used to deposit this every week.

According to Tim, when his grant finally came, it was a large lump sum and 'it just went straight to my mum because she'd worked to keep me there'.

His parents' economic support did not finish when Tim graduated, though its form was more indirect thereafter. When he left university, Tim successfully applied for a government Enterprise Allowance, which gave him a year's financial assistance to set up a small business. This was a market stall selling clothing, some of it hand-made, and some sold to specific orders. His parents again helped here, in two ways. First, they released some money which had been left for Tim as a trust in his grandmother's will, and he used this initially to buy stock.

Second, as a trained dress-maker, his mother's skills were very useful to him and she put herself at his disposal. Caroline was advising Tim on which clothing to purchase from manufacturers, how to price goods for sale, and also making clothing which he sold through his stall. Despite the fact that the business had not been wholly successful, Tim saw his mother's contribution as crucial in getting it going at all. Though he was very grateful to her, he presented their relationship as one which was strictly defined in economic terms, and from which she gained appropriate rewards.

Interviewer   Do you pay her?

Tim   We pay her by how long it takes her to do something.

Interviewer   We are interested in whether there are special terms between families on financial sorts of things. Do you pay her as much as you would someone else, or more, or . . .

Tim   We pay her, I'd say more than I would someone else because the work which she does for us is very, very good.

Caroline gave us a rather different account of the arrangement. Describing the clothes which she had made for Tim to sell she said:

Caroline   He gets the money for them. You know, he charges the shop price.

Interviewer   Yes. And he pays you?

Caroline   Oh yes. He'll say 'Here, that's for making that dress, mum.' It's not an hourly rate by any means but I do take it.

The two slightly differing accounts of the financial arrangements between mother and son are interesting here, reflecting the different ways in which they position themselves in relation to the commitment which Caroline was showing to securing her son's economic future. Caroline positions herself as a mother who is doing everything which she can to get her son established financially, and her work for him is really part of her continuing responsibility to him rather than a means to financial gain for herself. Thus she is quite happy for the pay to be 'not an hourly rate', in other words, that she does not actually get paid fully for the work which she does. On the other hand she says 'I do take it', indicating that she knows she needs to be careful not to move the relationship too far away from a business arrangement. For his part Tim is keen to emphasise the business element, saying that he pays his mother the rate for the job. Any other arrangement would rather jeopardise his adult status. As he puts it elsewhere in his interview:

Tim   I feel now that I'm 22 I'm old enough to look after myself really. I wouldn't say that I don't want to take any more off them. But I feel as if by *this* age I *should* be independent [pause]. I suppose in a way because I'm still near them I'm still linked to them. But I would never take any money from them. Like in the business I always pay my mum. [Emphasis in original]

In this family therefore we have an example of parents – especially a mother – who had taken significant economic responsibility for a son in early adult life, though the negotiation of the form which this should take was actually quite tricky. Though clearly regarding it as a part of continuing parental responsibility, she and Tim are both keenly aware that more is at stake simply than his economic position. It is clearly in Tim's material interests to go on accepting help from his parents; however, he does not want to because it would compromise his independence and his adult status. Even his present reliance upon his mother's expertise and labour to support his business is somewhat uncomfortable, hence his desire to define it purely as a business relationship and not a continuation of his economic dependence on his parents.

Taking this family as an example of one where parents do see themselves as retaining some responsibility for their son's financial status into adult life, on what kind of foundations was this responsibility based, and how had it come about? One important factor was that Caroline in particular saw herself as coming from a family whose members had a strong sense of commitment to each other, and an extensive history of mutual aid. She described her family as, 'very close [pause]. You kick one and they all limp [pause]. Now Lawrence's family are not quite so close.' Caroline saw herself continuing this in her relationship with her son. The point which we want to emphasise is that, in Caroline's eyes, she was not saying that *any* family would provide the kind of help which she had given Tim, that it is simply a 'natural' part of family life. Rather she sees it as a characteristic of *her* family to be a channel of mutual aid, a characteristic in which she took pride. We discuss a different example of mutual aid in Caroline's family in Chapter 2 and, certainly in relation to other kin groups in our study, they do represent a family whose members took a particularly strong view of their responsibilities towards each other.

Thus the kind of economic responsibility which Caroline accepted for her son cannot be understood fully without knowing the context of her wider kin relationships. It also cannot be understood without knowing something of the personal biographies of all the people involved. Lawrence and Caroline both had a strong sense that it was important to give Tim a better start in life than either of them had had. Lawrence seemed to have gone into his own father's business without much enthusiasm and did not want his own son to do the same. The way in which biographies get interwoven also comes through when we consider what implications their considerable assistance to Tim is likely to have for their future relationships. Caroline and Lawrence had spent much of their married lives fulfilling commitments to supporting one or other of their ailing parents on a daily basis. The first of these – Lawrence's father – had died just a few months before we conducted our interviews. As Caroline put it:

Caroline   We have lived here literally tied. We've just been saying, this is the first time in thirty years that we will be just us [pause]. Lawrence and I have never been able to go anywhere without telling somebody where we were going. If we wanted to go away for a weekend or something we had to make elaborate arrangements.

The experience of being highly committed to her own parents and parents-in-law led Caroline to say that she did not want Tim to feel tied in the same way by responsibilities to herself and Lawrence. Tim also felt that he would be less closely involved with his parents once he had left home and in a sense he was looking forward to that. However, his own view of his future relationship with them was coloured by aspects of his own biography and theirs. He had watched Caroline and Lawrence's strong commitment to the support of their own parents in old age and realised that there would be a very sharp contrast if he himself took no responsibility for them. In this context, he is aware that as an only child their interest is centred on him. In looking into his own future, he envisages moving to London, marrying at some stage and possibly having children himself. He sees this as a time when he would be much less involved with his parents than he is now, though in regular contact. However, looking further into the future, 'in my mid-thirties', he envisages a time when he might begin to feel a clearer sense of responsibility to his parents.

> *Interviewer*   In what sorts of ways do you think that [moving to London] would affect your relationship with your parents and the wider family?
> *Tim*   Well the ties will slowly start breaking I would think. The responsibility, well the responsibility won't be broken at all. There'll still be weekly contact by telephone or letters or whatever.
> *Interviewer*   What, you feeling responsibility to them or them to you?
> *Tim*   Them to me. I don't feel responsible to them at all really. [Laughs] Until my mid-thirties I probably won't do.

What comes across very clearly in this extract is the importance of time. Tim sees family responsibilities as varying over his life-time, rather than being fixed features of the scene. But time is important in another sense too. Responsibilities towards parents or children are not negotiated in a vacuum when a need arises, but are built upon a history of the relationship between parent and child, into which the biography of each gets incorporated and gives significance to the form which responsibilities might take. Tim anticipates that at some point he will take on an active responsibility for his parents, at least in part *because* he has seen them do it for their parents. He knows that it will be important for him to acknowledge that he does feel responsible for them, though he also knows that he will want to establish at a later stage precisely what form that responsibility will take. His parents seem also to have the same broad understanding of their future relationships, though neither they nor Tim seem to have a very clear idea of what it would mean for them in practice that he would take some responsibility for them in old age.

In discussing the Gardners, so far we have placed the emphasis on the private negotiations between the three parties, but there is also a public dimension to the way in which their relationships get shaped. Public norms about family responsibilities do have some relevance, but they are not rules which simply get 'applied'. Their importance enters the scene through a sense – conveyed especially by Caroline – that there is an external audience who observe what goes on and make judgements upon it. When she talks about going out to work to keep Tim at university she says:

> *Caroline* Me doing this for Tim is quite normal up here. You know you find that mothers are quite willing, perhaps not to make the sacrifice I made with every penny I earned [pause]. But there are other ladies. There were two in the place that I worked. One of them had two of her boys – but they were in a better position because they did get their grant straight away and she just helped with a contribution.

The picture which Caroline conveys here is being part of social world in which mothers make economic sacrifices to put their sons through higher education. She has obviously talked about it extensively with other women, and shared the details of their respective arrangements. She does not see it as a natural part of motherhood – by emphasising that 'it is quite normal up here' she implies that she believes that mothers elsewhere (perhaps outside the north west?) do *not* do it. But showing that she is willing to do this – indeed that she will go further than most and give 'every penny she earned' to her son – establishes her public identity as a generous and committed mother. The point is that she was not simply obeying the rules of motherhood and doing what was expected. She was doing *more* than could be expected and thereby gained the respect of other people. Her public identity, as well as her relationship with her son, was bound up in these negotiations.

Many points could be drawn out of this case study. However, since it is simply being used as a preliminary example here, we shall confine ourselves to a few which seem important to make at this stage. First, people do acknowledge responsibilities to kin but – in this example at least – they do not conceive of this as following rules of obligation. In this respect our survey data and our interview data point in the same direction, and underline the complexity of understanding these processes in the context of kin relationships in contemporary Britain.

Second, we think that the case which we have discussed does underline the importance of looking at the process of negotiation of responsibilities if we are to gain a full understanding of how they work in practice. Our survey data necessarily treat responsibilities in a static way, posing questions which have to be settled at one point in time. But in reality specific responsibilities emerge as part of longstanding relationships between the parties which have a past as well as a present, and anticipate a future. The past and the future are at least as important as the present in understanding how people come to accept family responsibilities.

Third, public norms about family obligations do get taken into account when people are negotiating their own responsibilities to kin, but again not in a straightforward way. People may be concerned about how their actions will appear to the outside world but this is not a matter of following the correct rules. It is more to do with constructing public images and personal identities.

CONCLUSION

We have tried to use this chapter to introduce our study of family responsibilities in several senses. First, we have been discussing the foundations of our work, especially the intellectual and political importance of studying these questions. Second, we have tried to introduce readers to the main features of our data set, to give a flavour of what it contains and what can be said about it.

Our main substantive point in this chapter concerns the central question of whether people in Britain in the late twentieth century do have a clear sense of family responsibilities and of what actions they imply. The simple answer to this is no. However we have also been able to point to some clues about how people do arrive at responsibilities and commitments in practice, and what significance these have. We have highlighted the importance of understanding processes and procedures; of looking at relationships between two people in the context of their family relationships as a whole; of understanding people's present actions in the light of their own biographies and those of other people; of looking at exchanges of assistance as a two-way process and seeing how people position themselves in relation to that process. These are all issues which we take up and examine further in the rest of the book.

2 Balancing responsibilities: dependence and independence

INTRODUCTION: THE IMPORTANCE OF KIN SUPPORT IN PRACTICE

In this chapter we begin our detailed exploration of how family responsibilities operate in practice. In the last chapter we argued that, at the level of publicly expressed norms, there are very few matters concerned with kin responsibilities on which there is clear agreement among a representative sample of the population. This might lead us to conclude that kin relationships are of little importance in contemporary Britain, indeed that the extended family has all but disappeared at least as a social support system – an argument which many other writers and researchers have addressed (Young and Willmott, 1957; Fletcher, 1966; Rosser and Harris, 1968; Firth et al., 1970; Morgan, 1975; Allan, 1985). However, it is dangerous to assume that beliefs expressed in a survey of this kind straightforwardly reflect what people actually do in their own families. The relationship between expressed beliefs and actions in practice is more complex than this in all areas of social life, family relationships included (see Finch, 1987b for further discussion).

The findings of our qualitative study suggest that, in practice, kin relationships *are* an important source of assistance to individuals, and for some people they are very important. We asked our interviewees, in a very open-ended way, whether there were examples in their own families of people helping each other and they offered us a large number. In Appendix C we have summarised some of the main patterns of giving and receiving assistance which we found in our qualitative data. Of course we need to be cautious about what we think these data can tell us about experiences of the population in general, as opposed to the experiences of individuals, where they have rich potential. Our qualitative study population was not designed to be a representative sample. Therefore we do not know if the patterns which we found among the eighty-eight people whom we interviewed would be repeated in a larger and a representative group. For example, by chance we could have selected a lot of people who have lent money to relatives, or rather few people who have cared for a sick person. So we cannot use the data from our study population to say *how common* it is to do either of these things. However, although we cannot generalise from their experience in that particular way, we can indicate what are the common or unusual experiences among *this group* of people – who do number eighty-eight, quite a large group by comparison with many intensive studies of family life. We shall be using the data from their interviews particularly to tell us something about *the range* of experiences which these people have had and therefore about a range of ways in which relatives do assist each other in contemporary Britain.

The data summarised in Appendix C give an overview – of the sketchiest kind – of what the experiences of our study population look like when they are added together. They show, for example, that almost everyone has either given or received financial help, though often the amounts of money passing between relatives were small. They show that about half the women – and only slightly fewer of the men – said that they had helped to look after a relative who was ill or incapacitated. They also show that about half the people in our study population have had experience of living in a household which contained an adult relative who was not part of a nuclear family. In all these three major categories – help with money, housing and personal care – experience of being involved in family assistance is therefore quite widespread among our study population, though of course simply adding together people's experience in this way masks wide variations in what this actually means, and especially in the demands which it made on the individuals involved. But our main point is that these are situations with which many people have some familiarity.

In addition to these, Appendix C documents a wide range of other types of assistance which relatives give each other – practical assistance, looking after young children, emotional support. The significance of these examples lies not so much in the number of people involved but in the wide range of examples which we are able to document. Family members do, it seems, support each other in many different ways when needs arise. The important question of how such assistance comes to be transacted is something which we address in later chapters.

On the question of *who* gets involved in such exchanges our data show a rather diverse pattern: under each type of support we have examples of assistance being given between cousins, aunts and nephews, grandparents and grandchildren, or in-laws. However it is also clear that, in the experience of our study population, it is more common for help to be given between parents and children. Since our survey data suggest that parents' responsibility to help their children is stronger than the reverse, it is interesting to find that this pattern is also reflected to an extent in the interview data. Table 2.1

Table 2.1 Examples of who gives help to whom (based on the data given in Appendix C)

	Parents to children	Children to parents	Other
Financial help	89	10	37
Providing a home*	25	18	8
Practical help	10	27	37
Emotional support	35	13	44
Totals	159	68	126

* This excludes 21 young adults who had never left the parental home, but might well do so.

summarises these patterns, for different types of support. We have excluded child care, on the grounds that it is unlikely to be given by children to their parents; similarly we have excluded personal care because it is more likely that older people rather than younger people will require this. The categories included in Table 2.1 are restricted therefore to types of help which, in principle, could pass either up or down the generations.

Table 2.1 shows that parent–child exchanges dominate over all others except in relation to giving practical help. Parents' support for their children is much more common than the reverse in relation to financial help and emotional support, and to a lesser extent in provid- ing a home. But in relation to practical help, we have more examples of children giving this to their parents than the other way round. We must underline that we are not claiming that these figures show the prevalence of such experiences in the population as a whole. They are simply the examples which our group of interviewees gave to us, and which reflect the balance of their experience. It is the meaning and the dynamics of these exchanges which was our main concern in our research, and upon which our discussion concentrates.

We shall be filling out the picture given in Appendix C as we move through our discussion in this and subsequent chapters. But in adding people's experiences together in this way, we run the risk of missing another important point. There is actually considerable diversity of experience among our study population in the extent to which they have been involved in giving or receiving any of the different types of help which we have mentioned. At one end of the spectrum are some people who seem to have been through practically the whole range. For example Sally Brown, a woman in her late thirties when we interviewed her, with two young children, at various times in her life had:

* received financial help from her parents to put her through a teacher training course, and then subsequently to buy her first house;

- moved back to live with her parents when she was unexpectedly widowed in her twenties;
- relied heavily on her parents' emotional support during the period following her bereavement;
- helped to nurse her mother through a terminal illness;
- received regular babysitting from her father;
- given practical help to a cousin who was caring for her own infirm mother; given practical assistance to a sister who was getting established with her own small business;
- given a temporary home to her father who was coming to terms with his own widowhood;
- anticipated that she would have her father to live with her at some stage in the future.

For Sally Brown, this list could probably be extended even further. For other people it would be very much shorter. At the opposite end of the spectrum we could place someone like Maureen Vickers, who was aged 65 when we interviewed her. She lived with her son, who was in his thirties, had never married and had always lived with his mother (one of the situations in which adults do share a home, though one which is relatively rare in our data set, as Appendix C shows). Apart from the mutual assistance between herself and her son, Maureen gave the impression of resolutely resisting any commitments to other relatives. Indeed before the interview started she said that she had 'no family' other than her son. In fact she had a sister, nieces and nephews in the south of England but she saw them rarely and felt no specific ties to them. She said, 'I never think of going down there and she never, well she never comes up here because I have no room for her.' Maureen also had had a brother who was now dead, but when he was alive she 'never saw him, never bothered with them'. She could give no examples of assistance passing between relatives and she positively disapproved of any financial assistance passing in families, and in this was very unusual in the context of our study population (see Appendix C).

If everyone had been like Maureen Vickers, we might be concluding that in practice kin are of little significance as providers of social support. However, we should also point out that Maureen had, in the past, fulfilled a very major commitment to caring for her mother in the last years of her life – indeed we used this example in Chapter 1. We have also noted that she and her son were heavily dependent on each other. Therefore it would be wrong to say that mutual aid between kin has been unimportant in her life. It has, however, been confined to parent–child relationships, which was not the case for most people in our study population.

So there were variations in our study population in the extent to which people were involved with kin. In some cases people simply did not have many relatives, but in other cases the variations cannot be explained so simply. Our subsequent chapters do address this issue, especially Chapter 3 where we examine how commitments to kin develop over time. However in general there would be few of our interviewees who would totally deny the importance of kin as a potential source of assistance. A common theme in our data set, which is reflected in a large number of interviews, is that people value the wider family group especially for its capacity to provide a network of support in crisis situations. The least that you can do for your relatives is to rally round in a crisis – this seems to be the touchstone of whether a family can really be said to 'exist'. The assistance given in this kind of situation may not necessarily be very demanding – though it can be so sometimes. At absolute minimum (the 'very least' you can do) it entails being a sympathetic listener and giving moral support when crises arise involving death, divorce, serious illness or some major life change. A small minority of our interviewees said that they would prefer to turn to friends for support in such crises but, for most interviewees who commented on this, kin would be the people on whom they would expect to rely for moral support. Indeed it felt like the essence of family life that you have people to fall back on in a crisis.

Where such crises generated practical needs, again it was seen as an absolute minimum that relatives should offer help, especially if this help was not too personally demanding. Though we were given a variety of examples, we noted that giving lifts in cars was mentioned by a number of people in this context. Also interesting is that several of those examples involved young men giving lifts in their car to a relative who needed to go on regular hospital visits, to someone who was temporarily incapacitated, or who had recently been bereaved. In these instances both the commitment and the inconvenience seemed fairly minimal, yet our interviewees thought it worth mentioning these to us as examples of assistance given and received. We think that they are indeed important – and their symbolic significance is at least as important as their practical value. In defining these as examples of kin support, our interviewees are telling us that their own family 'works' because it responds to members' needs. They are also telling us that young men, who otherwise may be rather little involved in exchanges of assistance, are not absolved completely.

These then are some of the main patterns apparent in our qualitative data set. We will be using it more extensively – along with our survey data – in this and subsequent chapters. In short it shows both the continuing significance of kin as people who provide assistance of various kinds, and also considerable variety in people's experience of giving and receiving such assistance.

GIVE AND TAKE IN KIN EXCHANGES

We see therefore that in practice many people do share mutual aid of various kinds with members of their kin group. However, at the level of publicly endorsed norms and beliefs, there is no obvious set of rules which indicates that any of us has a responsibility to give particular types of assistance to our relatives. The emphasis on procedural guidelines (rather than substantive rules) which emerged in Chapter 1, indicates the importance of focusing upon the *processes* through which help gets offered and accepted, given and received.

In much of the existing literature on kinship the concept of reciprocity is a key idea which is used in explaining the foundations of mutual aid in families. It refers to the way in which people exchange goods and services as part of an ongoing and two-way process. Receiving a gift creates the expectation that a counter-gift will be given at the appropriate time. Though reciprocity can take different forms, it is widely seen as being central to the dynamics of kin relationships (Finch, 1989: 162–7). In common usage, the idea that family life is essentially a matter of 'give and take' expresses the same idea while leaving unclear the crucial question of who should take what from whom, and in what circumstances. In the rest of this chapter we shall explore the dynamics of two-way exchanges as a way of developing an understanding of the underlying processes which lead one person to give help to another when a need arises.

Our survey data indicate that repaying favours done in the past is a potent idea at the normative level. This comes across clearly in one of our longer vignettes concerning the continuing relationship between a woman and her former mother-in-law after the younger woman's divorce. In the vignette, we built up a story in which the two women had a long history of mutual assistance and posed questions about whether this should continue despite the formal change in their relationship. We set out the question like this, inviting people to answer in three stages:

a. Jane Hill is a young woman with children aged 3 and 5. She was recently divorced. She wants to go back to work and she needs the money. But if she has a job she must find someone to mind the children after school. Her own family live far away but her former mother-in-law Ann Hill, is at home all day and lives nearby. Jane has always got on well with her former mother-in-law.
Should Jane offer to look after Ann's children?
b. Ann *does* offer to help and Jane goes back to work. Some years later Ann has a stroke and needs regular care and help in the home.
Should Jane offer to give up her job and look after her former mother-in-law?

c. Jane *does* give up her job. A year later Jane remarries.

Now that Jane has remarried, should she go on helping her former mother-in-law?

Why do you think she should go on helping/should stop helping?

In answering the first part of the question 87 per cent of our respondents said yes, Ann should offer to care for Jane's children. As our consensus baseline (see Chapter 1 for explanation) was 75 per cent for this question, this represents a notable measure of agreement. On the question of Jane giving up her job to care for Ann the proportion saying yes fell to 43 per cent with 41 per cent saying no. This split pattern of answers was similar to some other questions where we asked about a woman giving up a job to care for an elderly person. On the last part of the question 77 per cent said that Jane should go on helping her mother-in-law despite her own remarriage (again above our consensus baseline of 75 per cent).

Obviously there are a number of interesting issues raised by this pattern of answers, concerning the nature of in-law relationships and the impact of divorce upon them. We have discussed these in detail elsewhere (Finch and Mason, 1990c). The main point of mentioning this example here is because we believe that it shows the continuing strength of the principle of reciprocity. Even though the two women have had the formal structure of their relationship changed by divorce and then by remarriage, it appears that most of our survey respondents feel that their history of mutual aid gives them compelling reasons to go on helping each other. They have built up commitments which, we would argue, themselves provide the driving force for the relationship to continue. This interpretation is reinforced by the reasons which people gave us for their answers to the final part of the question, where many respondents emphasised that the relationship should continue because of the support that Jane and Ann had given each other in the past.

Thus, at the level of publicly expressed norms about family life, our survey population endorsed the principle of reciprocity. On the other hand they also gave us indications that the principle of reciprocity should not override everything. This is apparent where about half our respondents said that Jane should not give up her job to look after Ann. They were, as it were, drawing the line at that point. A similar message comes through in another vignette, where we asked if a grand-daughter should give up work to care for Mary Harper, her ailing grandmother. We built in the possibility that respondents would see this in the context of repaying favours done in the past, by indicating that the grandmother previously had paid the deposit to enable her grand-daughter to buy a house. However, even in these circumstances, only 29 per cent said that the grand-daughter should give up her job and 57 per cent said that she should not. Neither of these figures reaches our consensus baseline but it is interesting that twice as many people said that the grand-daughter should keep the job, as said that reciprocal responsibilities would require her to give it up. (There are also issues here about the circumstances under which women are expected to give up jobs, which we have discussed in Finch and Mason, 1990d.)

In the survey data therefore we find that most people do endorse the idea of repaying favours done and see this as an important principle in kin relationships, but acknowledge that there are limits to what can be expected as repayment. In these questions which we have discussed, the principle of reciprocity was endorsed equally strongly by women and men, and by younger and older respondents. The main variations in the way that people answered these questions concerned our respondents' own economic circumstances. We can identify a small group who seem to endorse the principle of reciprocity very strongly, by picking out just those respondents who said *both* that Jane Hill *and* the grand-daughter in the Harper vignette should give up their jobs to provide care for the elderly relative who had helped them in the past. There are 107 of them, about 10 per cent of our survey population. We looked at the characteristics of this group and found that the categories of respondents who were most likely to say that both women should give up their jobs were those whose own labour market position was relatively weak – people with no educational qualifications, or who fell in the lowest income band, or whose occupations put them in the lower social classes, using the Registrar General's scale. People who identified themselves as Christian (as opposed to having no religion) were also more likely to say that both women should give up their jobs to care for their elderly relative who had assisted them in the past. (These relationships are all significant at less than 1 per cent level.) It looks as if we are picking up here a reflection of people's views about the importance of a woman having a job rather more than variations in adherence to the principle of reciprocity. In general, therefore, our survey data offer no evidence that there are significant sub-groups of the population with distinctive beliefs about reciprocity. Certainly the factors of age and gender do not make any noticeable difference at this level of publicy endorsed beliefs.

So what about the principle of reciprocity in practice? Does it represent a significant part of the way in which people develop commitments to their own kin? Does it explain why some people get more involved than others in kin exchanges? And in what ways does the dynamic of gift and counter-gift actually work?

In examining our qualitative data on these issues we are going to argue that the dynamic of reciprocity *is* important in kin exchanges but that it works in specific ways. Central to our discussion of how reciprocity operates in practice is the concept of balance. We are going to argue that getting the balance right is a central part of negotiating responsibilities and commitments within kin groups. But the way in which 'balance' is calculated does not rely solely on the material value of the goods and services exchanged. A central theme in classic accounts of reciprocity is that exchanges of goods have a symbolic as well as a material value. Our analysis follows this theme, focusing particularly upon one aspect of symbolic value which is prominent in our data: the balance between dependence and independence. This is the key idea around which we develop discussion in the rest of this chapter. In particular we examine the processes through which individuals try to achieve 'the proper balance' in their relationships with kin, ensuring that no one becomes too frequently on the receiving end of assistance without also being in the position of a donor, and vice versa. Giving something in return enables the proper balance of dependence and independence to be maintained, and enables you to go on receiving.

These are the central ideas which we shall explore in the rest of this chapter. In order to highlight some of our key themes, we begin by discussing a case example. In this example, it is apparent that striving for a proper balance between dependence and independence is a crucial factor in shaping kin relationships over a long period of time. It also shows that personal costs can be entailed in trying to achieve a proper balance.

EXAMPLE: SARAH ALLEN'S RELATIONSHIP WITH HER PARENTS

When we interviewed her Sarah Allen was a woman in her late forties, living in a terraced house (which she owned) with her son Tim, who was 23 and about to begin a job as an executive officer in the Civil Service. Sarah herself had not been employed for several years although previously she had worked as a secretary. She had left her last job because she was suffering from depression. Sarah's parents were both still alive and they lived across the other side of the Greater Manchester conurbation. Sarah was seriously concerned about her father's state of health and her mother's capacity to cope. Although social services were involved with her parents, their situation caused her considerable anxiety and she visited them very regularly, taking a very complicated and lengthy journey involving several buses. Sarah had two older brothers, both of them married with grown-up children, both living nearer to her parents, both of whom had their own transport, but both of whom were less actively involved with their parents than was Sarah.

We are going to focus upon Sarah's relationship with her parents, in particular with her mother, about which she talked at length. Her predominant feeling about her parents at the time of interview was anxiety: 'they're hardly able to look after themselves but my mother won't admit it'.

This anxiety focuses particularly on her mother. Her father was showing clear signs of senility and the whole family found him very difficult. Her mother, however, had to manage him all day and Sarah was very aware that their relationship had never been an easy one, 'I suppose my mother has a lot of guts really because she's the one that's with my father all the time.' Though she admired her for her current fortitude, at the same time Sarah's own longstanding feelings about her mother were never far below the surface. She told us that their relationship had always been difficult and that her mother had always found fault with her. Despite her desire to give her parents support in the circumstances where they now found themselves, this dimension of their relationship still surfaced.

> *Sarah* If on a vulnerable day, if I'm tired or whatever, she starts on things that are kind of lashing out at old wounds. Well, I mean, really for me to suit her I would have to be an entirely different person.

If we just consider Sarah's present situation, we can see her trying to renegotiate her relationship with her parents in a way which changes the previous balance of dependence and independence. She wants them to accept her help in a way which would make them more dependent *on* her than they have ever been in the past – a redefinition which clearly her mother is resisting. Sarah's capacity to redefine the relationship to suit the changed circumstances is coloured by the history of her relationship with her mother. The personal animosity between them certainly is one aspect of that. But to understand fully the nature of Sarah's present difficulties with her parents, we need also to understand the way in which the balance of giving and receiving, of dependence and independence, had been negotiated in the past.

Central to this past history of the balance of responsibilities is a period when Sarah was a younger woman. She had gone to live in the United States when she was in her early twenties and was married to an American citizen. When that marriage ended, she returned to England with her son, who was then 5 years old. She went to live with her parents for about three years and clearly was quite heavily dependent upon them both for material and emotional support. Her mother also 'took over completely' the upbringing of Sarah's son. In a sense, her parents were put in a position where they accepted Sarah's renewed dependence on them, at a time when they might otherwise have expected her to be wholly independent.

Sarah says this was a very difficult period and ascribes some of the difficulties to her own inability to work out an independent lifestyle.

> *Sarah* I wasn't doing anything about getting out [pause] expecting to be rescued I think, by a knight in shining armour. But in the end it was my mother who did something about getting this house.

Her mother, having accommodated Sarah and her son for three years, took the initiative to move Sarah into her own house and found the money to do so. This appears to have been an attempt on her mother's part to redefine their relationship by making Sarah more independent of her. However, her mother kept control in important ways: by keeping actual ownership of the house in her own name for some years and by monitoring Sarah's activities quite closely, especially in relation to the care of her son. Sarah gives detailed descriptions from this period (which clearly were still vivid in her own mind) about incidents where, for example, her mother complained because she was not washing Tim's clothes properly. Sarah commented that she now understood a bit better than she did at the time how these situations arose, which often led to 'terrible rows'.

> *Sarah* I was reflecting on this, reflecting on the relationship, and I just happened to remember this – it was years before. And I thought: she manoeuvred me. It's as if she wants me to be incompetent, selfish, apparently either because that's the way she perceived me years ago and she can't do with perceiving me any other way. So she manipulates the circumstances so that I wind up appearing that way.

So, at the time we interviewed her, Sarah was struggling to redefine the relationship with her parents to take into account their apparent need to become more dependent upon her. This is a situation which no doubt many daughters have to face. Yet we cannot simply understand the situation in this family as 'an example' of the difficulties which both mothers and daughters experience in coming to terms with the dependency of the older generation. The distinctive features of Sarah's struggle were created by the history of *this* relationship – a relationship in which Sarah's mother had come to see herself as 'responsible for' Sarah in a strong sense. For her part, Sarah certainly felt a need to repay the considerable assistance which she had received in the past by helping her parents in old age. The strength of her commitment is demonstrated by the fact that she persevered in trying to help despite her continuing difficulties with her mother. However, Sarah's offering support was not sufficient – her parents also needed to be willing to accept it. In a sense, the same events which probably made Sarah more persistent in offering her help also made it more difficult for her mother to accept it. Because she had felt responsible for Sarah for many years, we can see that it would be especially difficult, in this case, for her to enter into a changed relationship in which Sarah became 'responsible for' her.

This example suggests that issues of dependency also are concerned with the exercise of power in family relationships. At least in Sarah's eyes, when her mother 'took responsibility' for Sarah and her son in the past she was also constituting her position as one in which she had considerable control –

her mother kept ownership of Sarah's house for several years, she monitored Sarah's activities closely, she 'manoeuvred' and 'manipulated the circumstances' of Sarah's life to produce the outcomes which she thought appropriate. There is a sense in which the concept of 'taking responsibility' for someone else necessarily implies that you have some control over their activities. Just as feminists have argued that women's financial dependency in marriage creates a situation in which women are subordinate to men, so Sarah's account of her dependency upon her parents demonstrates that she felt in a subordinate position, especially to her mother who apparently played the more active role. All this had happened many years previously. But in her current attempts to redefine their relationship so that her parents accept that *they* are the dependent ones, Sarah inevitably is facing her mother with a transfer of power and control. We did not interview her mother, so of course we cannot be sure how she sees the situation. But, on the basis of Sarah's account, the way in which the relationship between them has developed over time seems bound to make it very difficult to achieve an acceptable balance betwen dependence and independence in her parents' old age.

This case has unique features of course, and we are not claiming that it represents a common experience. We have used it here because it opens up some of the themes which are found, albeit in different forms, in other parts of our data set in relation to the balance of responsibilities. We see, for example, the interplay of material dependencies in other dimensions of the relationship between two individuals. What is at stake are personal and social identities, not just the exchange of goods and services. We can also see that these have a strongly gendered character – the issues over which Sarah and her mother had tangled for many years were matters distinctively concerned with the performance of women's domestic and family responsibilities. Yet despite the distinctive difficulties of this relationship, we can also see that the parties were striving to create a 'proper balance' in their relationship, which got negotiated and renegotiated over time as circumstances changed.

We move on now from this case example to look at our two data sets more generally, and to consider the processes whereby people try to achieve the right balance of responsibilities.

DIRECT REPAYMENT

The most obvious way in which a balance can be maintained in kin exchanges is to ensure that *the same* kind of assistance flows in both directions. Payment is made in the same currency, as it were. In that way no one gets into debt and the balance is kept. The 'currency' need not be money: it can entail exchange of goods, accommodation, labour and time. Our data make it clear that the scope for direct repayment is fairly limited, but that certainly it does occur.

Our interview data contain a number of examples where people try to achieve a proper balance in this kind of way. Relationships between people in the same generation predominated here: of a total of eighteen examples, eleven were between siblings, siblings-in-law or cousins. Indeed it seems particularly characteristic of sibling relationships that a debt should be repaid in the same currency. Both women and men talked about this form of reciprocal support, although the actual examples given reflected the different ways in which men's and women's lives are organised.

Our clearest examples of direct repayment fall into two categories. First were those where women shared child care arrangements. Appendix C shows the full range of child care arrangements reported to us by interviewees and it can be seen that, out of a total of forty-five examples, nine involved sisters or sisters-in-law looking after each others' children, mostly on an occasional basis and with husbands participating in the arrangements in one case. Examples involving sisters or sisters-in-law represented about half of the child care arrangements which we categorised as 'occasional' and in this sense they form the most characteristic type of 'occasional' child care arrangement. The most characteristic type of 'regular' child care arrangement, among our study population, was care by the child's grandmother.

In the examples where sisters or sisters-in-law provided child care for each other it was stressed that one woman could ask for her children to be minded if she needed this, in the knowledge that she would be able to repay with exactly the same favour in the future. This neatly solved the problem which we were often aware of when people talked about child care – that it is all too easy to ask a relative (even a mother) to mind your children too often. It is something where people commonly did see a real potential for the exchange to become unbalanced, whether they were potential donors or potential recipients. In these circumstances, sharing child care with a relative who herself has young children is the ideal solution, because it enables the balance to be maintained.

Second, several examples of direct repayment concerned money, mostly on a small scale. This might involve actually providing small amounts of money when a brother or sister was short, or sometimes in subsidising some activity directly, for example paying the entrance fee for a brother to accompany you to a club.

Appendix C documents different types of financial assistance from relatives which had been experienced by people in our study population – for example, money for housing, for travel, to support education or employment – and in each category almost every example entails money passing from older to younger generations. In general, therefore, our data confirm a pattern which emerges from other studies, that there is an expectation that money will pass 'down' the generations in families, and not be shared on a reciprocal basis (Finch, 1989). Children sometimes worry about this, and insist that they are receiving a loan which will be repaid, but parents mostly see a continuing responsibility towards their children in adult life, and do not expect to receive direct recompense.

However, in our category 'daily living expenses' the pattern is a bit different. Out of sixty-one examples, twelve are of brothers giving money to sisters or vice versa. Most of these examples are of people in their young adult years, but sharing these small sums of money is not confined to young people. One arrangement was described by various members of the Mansfield kin group, which comprised six adult siblings, all with their own children and separate households but mostly living within relatively easy reach of each other (see Appendix A for kin group details). As Kevin Ellis, who had married into the family, put it:

> *Kevin*   If one of the family wanted to go out and he phones up and says 'Well, we can't go out because I've got no money' or something, I mean any one of the family would turn round and say 'Oh well, we'll lend you some and pay us back when you can.' I think that happens quite a lot through the family [pause]. It's something that's always been taken for granted I think, if you've got it to lend. Because you always know you're going to get it back anyway and it works both ways, you know. They'll do it for you and you'll do it for us.

As is clear in this example, money has a currency value in the most literal sense and can be paid back directly either as a loan being discharged, or by means of giving the same amount on a different occasion. Indeed these two forms of paying back may well be difficult to distinguish in practice.

Direct exchanges – whether of money or child care or anything else – are the most literal expression of the importance of keeping the balance between giving and receiving. The essence of these direct exchanges is that they do not create any sense of one person's being dependent upon another. They often involve precisely the same 'good turn' being done but at a different point in time. This seems to be a strategy particularly prominent in relations between people of the same generation. In most of the examples described, the type of help given was relatively undemanding and the timescale of repayment was quite short. This was not necessarily the case with more indirect examples of 'paying back', to which we now turn.

INDIRECT REPAYMENT: NEGOTIATING RATES OF EXCHANGE

There are two rather different senses in which exchanges of assistance between kin can be 'indirect'. In the first type of indirect exchange, two individuals exchange goods or services with each other, but different types of assistance flow in each direction: one gets child care, the other gets help with decorating, for example. In the second type of indirect exchange, there are more than two people involved: A receives assistance from B, but 'pays back' to C.

We shall deal with each of these in turn. The first type of indirect exchange is, as the American sociologist Alvin Gouldner (1973) put it in his discussion of reciprocity, 'tit for tat' rather than 'tat for tat'. Most forms of exchange are like this, he argues. This immediately raises the potential problem of agreeing on the right 'currency' for the exchange. There is no obvious way of determining how much practical help would repay a parent for lending you the deposit on a house, for example, or whether taking your mother to live with you when she is old is equivalent to the child care which she provided when your children were young. However, if the principle is important that one party should not become too dependent upon the other, then it is important to find some way of 'counting' equivalence.

In our data set we have thirty-two fairly clear examples of exchanges of this sort of indirect exchange – that is, where our interviewees gave some indication that *they* saw a particular example of assistance as part of a pattern of ongoing mutual support. Unlike our examples of direct repayment, most of these examples of indirect repayment involved people in different generations, half of them being between parents and children. The gender balance of these indirect exchanges seems a little different from the more direct examples, especially those which concerned money. In about half the cases (seventeen in total) both parties are women. In most of the rest, at least one of the parties was a woman. We have very few examples of indirect exchanges of assistance between two men, the clearest of which we discuss in some detail below (see: John Green and his grandchildren).

Again in contrast with our earlier examples, sometimes very significant forms of assistance were being repaid. It is also notable that, though some repayments were concurrent, in a number of cases the timescale of repayment was over many years. For example, Jane Ashton's step-father had provided regular child care for Jane's youngest child so that she could go out to work. Jane helped him in a variety of practical ways and fifteen years later she was setting up arrangements for him to move into her home at the point when he died. In another example, Marion Smith had supported her sister emotionally and practically when she went through the very traumatic experience of her husband being murdered. Giving emotional support at a time of bereavement is not uncommon in our data set. Appendix C shows that, out of forty-nine examples of people giving emotional support to a relative when specific events occurred (as opposed to doing this on a regular basis), fifteen involved a bereavement. However, the particular circumstances of Marion Smith's sister made the support which Marion gave very significant. In return, and several years later, she had felt able to ask her sister to lend money to assist with the purchase of a house. This is the only example which we have of such a loan between siblings, since financial help with housing is otherwise almost exclusively confined to parents helping their children. However, in this case, it would appear that the scale of emotional and practical support which had been given in the past made it possible for Marion to ask for a type of financial assistance which otherwise is rare between people of the same generation.

This example brings into focus the question of rates of exchange, and how they operate in these indirect examples. How is the 'value' of one form of help calculated, so that it can be repaid on an appropriate scale in a different form? We are going to explore the issue of rates of exchange by considering three examples, each of which highlights different issues. These cases are not intended to be 'representative', but they have been selected to cover a range of rather different experiences and situations. Between them they enable us to draw out some analytical points about negotiating rates of exchange which would apply more widely in our data set. We will present each example descriptively and then discuss them in relation to each other.

Example 1: John Green and his grandchildren

This example concerns the relationship between John Green and his grandchildren, especially one grandson. This case is unusual in our data set, since we have very few examples of clear, reciprocal responsibilities being built up between two men. John was in his seventies when we interviewed him and, although not in very good health himself, was heavily committed to caring for his mother-in-law who had lived with his wife and himself since they married ten years previously. John had been married before and widowed at quite a young age, subsequently bringing up the only child of this first marriage. His son now had three children, a daughter and two sons, one of whom was married with a young baby. John defined his son, grandchildren and great-grandchild as 'his family' and saw it as his responsibility to assist them where he could. Most of the examples of assistance which he gave us were financial, for example, when the great-grandchild was born, he had offered to take on full responsibility for buying all the clothes needed as the child grew up.

John's grandchildren, especially one unmarried grandson, gave his grandfather quite significant practical assistance round the house and garden whenever it was needed. Of itself this is not very remarkable. Appendix C shows that most of our examples of giving domestic and practical assistance of this type involve younger people helping older relatives. What is distinctive about this case is the context in which such help was given. Both John and his wife had been in professional occupations and were comfortably off financially. John's assets were to pass to 'his family' on his death and his grandchildren knew that they were going to be major beneficiaries. As a result, John felt able to call on his grandchildren's practical assistance as of right, in advance repayment for the financial help which they would receive from him. John explained his view of the implicit bargain with his grandchildren in this way:

> *John* I've got two grandsons and quite frankly I *expect* of them, and I'm not going to be surprised because I expect it. I'll say 'Look, I've done for you, now you can do something for me.' And I know that they won't have to be asked. So they'll know, the two of them you know. The bread's coming back, sort of thing [pause]. I expect them to come down and keep the garden in order and, er, possibly repair a few things under my supervision [laughs] and that sort of business. I don't intend to just sit back and say 'get on with it'.
>
> *Interviewer* No.
>
> *John* I've got to have my supervisory capacity otherwise it's not going to be any good to me. So it's got to be a partnership in that respect you see.

It seems that the grandchildren themselves were very aware of this bargain and one of them, who was clearly something of a favourite, was able to mention it openly though in a joking way, according to this exchange which John reported:

> *John* This boy Peter, he'll come here and on one occasion he says 'You know grandad when you push off' he says 'you can leave me this house. I rather like it. Yes, I like it. I think you had a bit of taste when you . . .'. He'll come down here, you know Peter, the middle one and 'Hello Peter, what do you want? What are you here for?' 'I just thought I'd come round and see how my property's getting on.' He's very pert but he's a good lad. If I get on the phone and say 'Peter, so and so, I want a bit of a lift with so and so.' 'Yes. When?'

Example 2: Jane Smith and her husband's kin

Our second example concerns the relationship between Jane Smith and her husband's kin, centred on relationships with her mother-in-law. Jane was a woman in her thirties with two young children. Neither she nor her husband were in paid work but their financial circumstances were not as stretched as they might have been because Jane's own mother, who had a private income, helped them regularly. Jane's mother-in-law had few financial resources and sometimes ran out of money completely, at which point she would come and stay in Jane's household and live on their resources for a while. Another indirect beneficiary was Jane's sister-in-law, who apparently expected Jane to drive her mother to visit her. Jane was therefore in the middle of a rather complex web of financial and other dependencies which inevitably were rather difficult to manage at times.

As Jane expressed it to us, a particular focus for dissatisfaction was the use of her car.

> *Interviewer* Do you have quite a lot of contact with her [your mother-in-law]?
> *Jane* Yes. Well we ... of her children we're the only ones with a telephone and a car [laughs].
> *Interviewer* Oh right.
> *Jane* So we get called upon frequently for ... well if she wants to come down and see us, or wants to go and see her other daughters, she calls us [laughs].
> *Interviewer:* And you take her over do you?
> *Jane* Yes well it's fairly local. She comes and stops here quite often if we need a babysitter.
> *Interviewer* Oh that's handy.
> *Jane* Occasionally yes, yes [pause] I get a bit cross. With one daughter she tends to use us rather a lot. I don't like that.
> *Interviewer* What – do you mean not sort of pulling her weight? with her mother?
> *Jane* Well it's difficult because she hasn't got transport. But she's working and we're not. She just takes it for granted sometimes that we'll pick her up and take her there, take her anywhere, and then drop her off home again.

Jane makes it clear here that there is *some* element of reciprocity in this relationship, in that her mother-in-law will babysit for them, but that this is *not enough* to repay the expectations that Jane's car will be available for her mother-in-law's use. Further, she resents the fact that her sister-in-law can call upon the use of her own car, without apparently reciprocating at all. In this instance the rate of exchange is unsatisfactory to one of the parties creating, from Jane's point of view, an inappropriate level of dependency over matters of transport. Jane is also left feeling that she is being 'used' by her mother-in-law and her sister-in-law.

Example 3: Caroline Gardner and her cousin

Our third example concerns Caroline Gardner, whose relationship with her son we discussed in Chapter 1. Here we are using data on the relationships between Caroline's own kin from her family of origin. In describing her kin group to us, Caroline presented them as unusually close, with complex intertwined patterns of practical assistance. She gave a number of examples of assistance which passed between aunts, uncles and cousins in her kin group, as well as between closer relatives. Apart from moral and emotional support at times of crisis, these examples all concerned practical assistance based upon the expertise of different relatives and Caroline insisted that it all took place on the basis of exchange: 'no money changes hands'. On the basis of Caroline's account the Gardners certainly fall at one end of the spectrum of kin groups represented in our study, especially in relation to sharing practical assistance. They also are one of two or three families who routinely mentioned aunts, uncles and cousins.

The example which we are going to use here concerns the relationship between Caroline and her husband Lawrence on the one hand and Rose, a female cousin of Caroline's, a woman in her sixties who had lived alone for many years. Caroline was very friendly with her and they saw a lot of each other. Rose had a three-piece suite which needed recovering and this was clearly a job which Lawrence Gardner could easily have done, as he was a self-employed upholsterer. As Caroline saw it Rose certainly could not afford to pay to have this job done outside the family because 'she only has a widow's pension'. However, Rose was reluctant to allow Lawrence to do the job for no payment. She clearly was concerned that assistance of this kind, if translated into money terms, would be 'too much' – more than the normal kind of help which flowed backwards and forwards in her kin group. If she accepted this help from Lawrence, the relationship between them would become unbalanced. Thus Rose entered into a very elaborate arrangement for 'paying back' which indicates how important it was that she did not get into a situation of inappropriate dependency upon Caroline and Lawrence. The opportunity to devise this arrangement arose because it was her custom to visit them once a week and have a meal with them.

> *Caroline* What happens is she [Rose] does my windows and . . . this'll sounds daft on your tape [laughs] . . . she wants her suite recovering and

knows it'll cost too much. So she cleans my windows and she'll do the ironing or whatever tomorrow and I'll put three pounds in a tin. She says, when there's enough in the tin Lawrence can recover her suite [laughs]. So there you are.

Interviewer Oh how interesting. How interesting.

Caroline She won't take the money off me, I can't give her money. I buy her dress lengths and make them up if she wants blouses. She'll take those off me but she won't take money. But . . .

Interviewer No. But equally she won't let your husband do the suite because that would be too much.

Caroline No. She wouldn't let him do that. So she said . . . we've got an aunt coming in September to stay. She sleeps with our Rose because she's got room [pause] And she wanted it recovering and she said 'Will I have enough money for September?' I said 'Look. If you've not, we'll do it for you anyway and you can work it off!' [laughs]. Isn't it awful?

This example is a rich one in relation to the issues which we are developing in this chapter. Caroline Gardner indicates that rates of exchange *are* of considerable importance in her family. Yet if this becomes too explicit, the processes of negotiation break down. In her own account she is making them sound explicit and so she distances herself from this by ending up laughing and saying 'Isn't it awful?'

At the same time, it is clear that Rose has a finely tuned sense of what constitute appropriate rates of exchange, coupled with a strong desire to ensure that the balance of her relationships is kept even. Her scheme for exchanging her own labour for that of her cousin's husband was made difficult by the fact that she wanted the exchange to be equivalent in financial terms, yet the *actual* transfer of money would contravene the customs of a family in which money never changes hands. The indirect exchange of equivalent services was arranged very literally, by calculating it in financial terms but placing money in a tin rather than handing it over. Caroline, as the person with potentially more to give, makes it clear that she can see the ludicrous side of this, but understands the reasoning which goes behind it and therefore will play the game on her cousin's terms.

Negotiating rates of exchange

By considering these three examples together, we can make a number of points about indirect exchanges and the processes by which they are negotiated. First and most obviously, it is often a very complex matter to arrive at an understanding of equivalent exchanges, which both parties see as appropriate, and which will not leave one party in the position of a net giver or a net receiver. Jane Smith clearly had quite a different concept of this from her mother-in-law and sister-in-law. Caroline Gardner and her cousin also had rather different concepts, in that Caroline would have been happy to settle for terms which were less advantageous to herself.

Second, the problem of not becoming too dependent on relatives is an ever-present worry for some people but apparently not for others. For Rose it was a major concern that, in negotiating appropriate rates of exchange, she should maintain a proper balance of dependence and independence. In sharp contrast, John Green saw no practical danger of the balance shifting so that he became too dependent. He felt that *anything* which his grandchildren might do for him could be seen as a right rather than a favour, given their position as his heirs.

What might make the difference between these two cases? Gender could certainly be one factor. John Green's lack of concern about being perceived as too dependent may simply be a man's insensitivity to that possibility. One could argue that men's lives – especially those of men like John who have had responsible jobs – generally are not organised in such a way as to put them in dependent positions, and therefore they are less attuned to this possibility in old age. By contrast, women are more likely to have experience of being dependent upon other people at many points in their lives – as wives, as mothers of young children needing some support, as people who cannot earn high enough wages to support themselves in full financially.

This explanation does fit the cases which we have used here, but looks less straightforward when we consider our data set as a whole. We have at least one case of an elderly man, John O'Malley, who apparently *was* very concerned about becoming too dependent on his daughter Jill. He had contracted multiple sclerosis and already relied on his wife quite heavily for practical assistance. He talked with considerable anxiety about the possibility that she would die before himself, leaving his daughter to take on the responsibility for an infirm father who could not be of any practical assistance to her – a responsibility which she expressed herself very willing to shoulder, in her own interview. This case is striking because there was a financial consideration of a similar type to that in the Green family. The O'Malleys were also secure financially and Jill was their sole heir. They had already given Jill's husband substantial financial help in his business. Yet for John O'Malley, unlike John Green, the financial support both given and to come did not counteract his concern about getting into a situation where he was receiving more than he could give. The most obvious contrast between the situations of the two elderly men is that John O'Malley, because of his physical condition, had already experienced a degree of practical dependency which was not part of John Green's experience. In a sense, therefore, his case strengthens our argument about the experience of gender as a factor in attuning people to the possibility of becoming too dependent. On the whole it is women rather than men whose lives are lived in ways which give them experience of dependency, but some men do have such experiences. Where they do, it would seem that this can sensitise them to the possibilities of imbalance in family relationships in ways which otherwise are more characteristic of women.

Our third and final point about these examples of indirect exchange concerns the exercise of power in this type of negotiation. It appears that the capacity to dictate the rates of exchange does not always rest with the person who – to an outsider – is in the most powerful position. In John Green's case, he took that right on the basis of the financial power which he held. But in the other two cases, the person with less to give appears to have been the one who successfully dictated the terms. Rose was able to insist on the terms in which she was going to engage in exchange of assistance with Caroline Gardner and her husband. In this instance it was relatively easy for her to accede to Rose's terms which, although looking slightly ludicrous, were nevertheless favourable to Caroline. Jane Smith however, despite apparently being in the more powerful position in that she had control of the car, was unhappy about the terms of exchange which her in-laws had succeeded in imposing and felt exploited as a consequence.

In understanding the difference between John Green and the other two cases, again gender may well be an important factor. As a man, indeed as a man who had worked in responsible jobs all his life, it probably came quite naturally to John to exercise the power over his grandchildren which their financial relationship to him apparently conferred. Certainly his reference to retaining a 'supervisory' role over the assistance which his grandchildren gave him seems to be a characteristically male form of relationship. For John, it drew explicitly on his experience of his working life, where his interviews make it clear that he did exercise supervisory authority over other people and that he took pride in doing so. Few women have such experiences to draw on and to bring into the way they shape their family relationships. This is one reason why it is difficult to imagine a parallel example in which a woman places herself in the position, not only of requiring assistance, but also of supervising how it is carried out.

In summary, it is apparent from these examples of indirect exchange that the idea of achieving a 'proper balance' is a very prominent consideration. We have used the metaphor of 'rates of exchange' as a way of discussing this, but it is important not to take it too literally. People are not simply trying to estimate the material value of goods received or labour performed in order to set the one against the other. It is more a question of deciding what is to *count* as enough to balance out one exchange against another – enough, that is, to ensure that one person is not *perceived* as being too dependent. There are no simple rules for calculating this. Indeed what counts as 'enough' may well vary from one family to another, and from one situation to another in the same family.

Despite the importance of the principle of reciprocity in the examples which we have discussed so far, it would be inaccurate (at least in terms of our data) to see absolutely all assistance in kin groups as locked into a logic of paying back which requires very fine calculations. In turning to the other type of indirect exchange, we move into territory where this logic operates rather differently, and in some ways is less prominent.

INDIRECT EXCHANGE: GENERALISED RECIPROCITY

We move on now to the other type of indirect exchange, where repayment is not straightforwardly between two individuals. The 'paying back' involves a third party, possibly more than one. In these situations the process of negotiating the balance between dependence and independence is diffuse and involves a number of individuals.

In existing literature on kin relationships, especially anthropological literature, these issues are conceptualised through the concept of 'generalised' reciprocity, which is contrasted with 'balanced' reciprocity and is said to be particularly characteristic of kin relationships. In its simplest form, balanced reciprocity implies direct repayment between two individuals on an equivalent scale. The concept of generalised reciprocity, by contrast, denotes circumstances in which a fairly immediate counter-gift is not expected, or may not be expected at all. There is simply the expectation that repayment will be made at some point, possibly to the same person but also possibly to a third party (Sahlins, 1965; Lévi-Strauss, 1969; Finch, 1989: Chapter 5). Alvin Gouldner, commenting on this phenomenon in American society, calls this type of reciprocity 'an all-purpose moral cement' which binds the parties together by creating a sense of indebtedness, and locks individuals into a set of relationships which have a diffuse and generalised expectation that people will reciprocate (Gouldner, 1973).

We shall consider examples of generalised reciprocity under two headings. First, there are instances where people feel an obligation to 'pay back' the support which they have received themselves, by giving the *same kind* of help to a third party. In our interview data, we have twelve examples of a person talking about this kind of exchange. In most of them the person who feels the pressure to pay back to a third party is talking about repaying the support which they received from an older generation, by giving similar assistance to the generation younger than themselves. The *form* of the exchange remains the same (older generations support younger ones in very similar ways), but the *individuals* who occupy the positions of giver and receiver change over time, as they move through their life courses.

A case typical of these twelve is Jill Archer, the daughter of John O'Malley whom we mentioned in the previous section (see Appendix A for details of this kin group). She typifies this form of exchange in the way she presents her relationships with her parents and her children, although she is unusual in that the actual amounts of money at her disposal were greater than for most of our other respondents. Jill was married to a veterinary surgeon. She worked full-time in her home caring for her four children – who were aged between 6 and 19 when we interviewed her – and in supporting her husband's work. She was an only child and had received significant financial and practical support from her parents in the past. The most substantial example – and it was one which all our interviewees in this family talked about – was a gift of £10,000 (at mid-1970s prices) from Jill's parents to her husband, to enable him to buy into a partnership in a veterinary practice. This is one of a total of ten examples which we have where financial support was given to a relative to help establish or sustain a business venture (see Appendix C) but it was also the single largest sum mentioned to us.

In discussing relationships across the generations in her family, Jill talked about her willingness to give money to her children – substantial amounts if necessary – to support their various activities in adult life, and linked this with the fact that she had received generous financial help from her own parents.

Interviewer With things like, say gifts of money to Shula, do you think that you would feel in years to come you'd like her to offer to pay it back, even though you weren't giving it to her as a loan?
Jill No, no. It's only money. But it's alright for me to say that because I'm secure. And that's what it is – it's only money. And I've had it freely given to me. My parents are *totally* generous.

Reflecting similar reasoning, though on a different scale of financial assistance, another of our interviewees, Tilly Trotter, told us that she tries to give her adult daughters financial help whenever she can, just as her mother did for her.

Tilly She [my mother] were fabulous. And I've tried to do that with my girls.
Interviewer Have you?
Tilly Yes, I've tried to do exactly the same. Well I've not tried – I've *done* it. It's come natural, you know. The other night [one daughter] [pause] knocked on the door and 'Mum, have you enough? I'm just a bit stuck for my electricty and gas.' 'There you are.' She has it – which my mother did for me.

Both the Jill Archer and Tilly Trotter cases are about repayment of money across generations, and both concern mothers and daughters. About half of the twelve cases which we have categorised in this group would fit this description. Rather different from these were three cases which were distinctive in that they concerned the migration of members of the family from one country to another, where support from other kin – usually those who had already migrated – was a significant way of facilitating these moves. The assistance could come in various forms including money. It involved reciprocal assistance across generations and was not confined to parents and children.

One of these cases came from an interview with a man of Asian descent, another from a young woman of Caribbean descent and the third from Paul Bailey, who had been brought up in Belfast. Paul's account of the importance of repaying the assistance which he himself had received was explicit, as were the accounts of the other two respondents who discussed migration. As a younger man, Paul had received help from an uncle to assist his migration to the United States (where he did not stay). Later he settled in England, and felt that he wanted to repay the help from his uncle by giving similar assistance to his own nephew when the occasion arose. The young nephew was living in Belfast and, in Paul's eyes, was in a rather vulnerable situation in a violent city. Paul was clear that he felt a responsibility to help his nephew settle in England.

> *Paul* I wanted to go to America once and my uncle Jack [pause] he works on the boats and he sent my fare to go to America and he also got me a job. He only knew me as a young boy, you know, he didn't know me as a man. He just took me over on the strength of family. He was really nice.
>
> *Interviewer* Do you think that most families are like that or do you think it's unusual?
>
> *Paul* I think so, yes. Same as Micky you know. When I, when I brought my brother's son over – we didn't really know what Micky was like. We knew him as a young boy but, you know, he was 17, 16 when he was with us – a young man. I was just taking him over because I knew he was my brother's son.

It is interesting that the three cases in our data set concerning migration come from people whose origins are in very different parts of the world. It appears that we are not talking about a phenomenon located in Indian culture, Irish culture or whatever, but picking up patterns of assistance which can occur widely in situations where it is fairly common to try to migrate for economic reasons (Grieco, 1987; Finch, 1989: 20–1). In these situations, the kin network appears to be drawn in quite extensively. Assistance seems to be given simply, as Paul Bailey put it, 'on the strength of being family'. These cases seem to come close to Gouldner's description of generalised reciprocity as a form of indebtedness which acts as an 'all purpose moral cement' which binds whole, large kin groups together. However, in our own data set this seems to be distinctive to the situation of migration. In other examples of paying back to a third party, more typically the exchanges are between parents and children across three generations, but do not extend more broadly.

We turn now to consider a different group of cases, where the repayment comes in the form of help of a *different kind*, but again to a third party. These examples are obviously much more diffuse and our interviewees did not normally present them explicitly as 'paying back'. We have included those cases in which there seems to be at least some evidence that the participants thought of their actions in this way, but there are probably many more of a less explicit kind in our data set. The clearest examples of this form of indirect exchange come from that minority of interviewees whose lives seem to be organised around kin relationships more significantly than others, and who presented their families as units where a lot of mutual support passes on a routine basis. In such families, one can trace patterns of assistance which seem to be based upon a generalised expectation that people will do good turns for each other on a regular basis. In other families, it is much more difficult to trace these more diffuse types of generalised reciprocity.

The Jacksons are one of our kin groups (see Appendix A) where this more diffuse version of generalised reciprocity seems prominent. This was a family in which the parents and their three adult sons (of whom we interviewed two) all seemed to see themselves as locked into a set of kin relationships in which mutual aid was a regular expectation. In interviews with different members of this family, we were able to document various different types of assistance flowing in all directions: financial help, emotional support, child care, practical assistance, personal care. One of the sons, Robert, who was in his thirties and who was our first contact in this family, said that his family was 'second to none' for giving each other mutual support and they obviously all took great pride in this.

Although the most regular flows of assistance were between the parents, children and children-in-law, the wider kin network was also included in a more muted form. The mother, Mary Jackson was heavily involved in giving regular practical and personal assistance to an elderly uncle and two elderly aunts who lived in the neighbourhood, as well as being available for any relative to call on in a crisis. Her husband and children were also drawn into this wider enterprise. For example, Robert told us that he was always called upon even by quite distant relatives when someone had died, to help with and advise upon practical arrangements. He was seen as being particularly suited to this because he had worked as a police officer for part of his life. He told the story this way in relation to the recent death of one of his great uncles:

> *Robert*   Well my Auntie Ethel and my mother and myself, we all shot over [to the hospital] the day he died. We all jumped into my car. As I said to you before, when it comes to death, it's me.
> *Interviewer*   You're the expert [laughs].
> *Robert*   This is what happened. When it came to the death, it was down to me to give advice and sort things out. My mother said, 'What about funeral arrangements Auntie Ethel, what do you want us to do?' And she said, 'Well Robert, what *do* you do?' [pause]. I sorted everything out and my Auntie Ethel did nothing, and my mother did nothing. There was nothing to do. It had all been sorted. It was down to me again. Death is Robert, you know [laughs].

In the accounts of the Jackson family, and others like them, one certainly gets a feeling of 'generalised indebtedness' being an important facet of family relationships and the foundation of much of the assistance which passes between kin, especially perhaps of smaller-scale assistance. We should emphasise again, however, that we think that there is a minority of kin groups to which this applies – certainly this is so within our data set. The families in which we can identify it most clearly – the Jacksons, the Mansfields and the Gardners (see Appendix A for details) – are all kin groups where most of the key members have been geographically mobile over short distances only, where there is a considerable amount of regular contact between kin, and where most members of the kin group have working-class occupations (typically 'respectable' working class). However, we have other kin groups in our study which apparently fit these same criteria, but where we do not get the same sense that 'generalised indebtedness' characterises their relationships. So the nature of kin relationships is not straighforwardly explained by factors such as geographical closeness, though they play some part.

In those situations where we can identify these diffuse forms of generalised reciprocity, there is another important feature. It seems that the impulse to 'pay back' is rather more muted than in other forms of exchange which we have discussed. By and large people do not seem to be overtly concerned about keeping tally of whether they are net givers or net receivers in the kin group as a whole. Although there may be some feeling that 'it all evens out in the end', the emphasis is much more upon everyone being prepared to share with others what talents and skills they have. There apparently is considerable tolerance for situations where some people are net receivers. It appears that this does not significantly threaten the balance between dependence and independence for any individual member of the kin group.

This tolerance of imbalance within the kin group as a whole is made explicit by Caroline Gardner, whose family was one of those which was extensively involved in sharing practical assistance. In answering a question about whether people ever worried that someone was being given a lot of help but not giving very much back, she said, 'Er not really, no. We must be well adjusted.' Caroline then went on to describe the help given recently to her cousin Rose, by a number of her kin as well as herself. Over one weekend various members of the family had got together and cleaned, repaired and decorated a flat which Rose was going to move into, laid carpets and bought new furniture for her. She also was receiving assistance with gardening over a longer term, and various members of the family tried to subsidise her financially in appropriate ways. When she had finished describing all this, Caroline said:

> You see what she does, now that she's 60, she babysits. If there's a dance on and one of her brothers has got children [pause] if they know they're not going to be back till 4 o'clock she goes to sleep, which is how she pays back.

Although (as we noted above) there is no obvious currency in which one type of assistance can be repaid by another, it seems clear that in this case Rose was a net receiver of support from her relatives. This seemed to present no apparent problems at this level of assistance within the kin group as a whole. But if we compare that with another situation concerning Caroline and Rose – which we discussed in the previous section – some interesting contrasts emerge. In relation to negotiations over re-covering Rose's three piece suite, there was a danger that the pattern of exchanges between two parties – Rose on the one hand, Caroline and her husband on the other – would become notably imbalanced. It went beyond the normal type of assistance which was exchanged and Rose was *very* concerned about paying back and was quite precise about her calculations. However, when it came to the normal pattern of exchanges within this family, Rose's position could easily be accommodated. It seemed to be enough that she was *willing* to give as well as to receive and that she actually did *what she could*. Apparently no one thought of her as 'the kind of person' who tried to avoid giving or repaying, and this was very important.

Linking this with our discussion of maintaining the balance of dependence and independence, it could be argued that the normal pattern of support within this kin group did not leave Rose in danger of appearing to be 'too dependent' on any single individual. She received a small amount of assistance from a number of people and thus was unlikely to become over-indebted to any of them. The fact that she clearly received more than she gave in relation to setting her up in a new flat, could be accommodated quite easily. Moving house is something that happens to a lot of people, and Rose could quite easily think of herself as on the receiving end now, but likely to be one of the donors in the future. The family was simply 'rallying round' to help someone who happened to need it at this particular point in time.

So in these specific situations, in the minority of families where there is a pattern of everyone 'rallying round' to give practical assistance when it is needed, it seems that some imbalance of dependence and independence can be tolerated quite readily. This seems to be characterised by a view that everyone *would* do what they could for their family, even though they may not be equally able to provide support at particular times. A crucial difference between this situation and all the others which we have discussed is that there is *no single individual* upon whom someone like Rose becomes dependent. Therefore there is no one to whom she is in danger of becoming subordinate. Unlike all the other cases which we have discussed, this form of exchange, and the type of indebtedness which it creates, does not imply putting yourself under someone else's control.

CONCLUSION

We began this chapter by noting that kin relationships do seem to be an important source of assistance in a range of situations where a person needs some practical or financial help, though there is also considerable variation in different people's experience of this. We have shown that this cannot be explained simply by the idea that people follow well understood rules of obligation or duty towards their relatives.

We have explored the idea of reciprocity as one way of understanding processes of exchange within kin groups – indeed the common way in which academic writing has tried to address these issues. By looking at our survey data, we found that reciprocity is a principle to which most people clearly give assent at the level of publicly expressed norms and beliefs. However, these data also show that, for most people, there are limits to reciprocity – or at least there are limits to what can be expected as repayment for favours done. When we look at what happens in practice in family life, the principle of repayment also seems to be important, but it is seldom straightforward to apply. There are some circumstances, we have argued, where repayment can be direct and in the same currency. But in most cases people are engaged in repaying one type of help with a different type of help, so the question of what counts as appropriate repayment is much more complex.

We have argued that the key to understanding the processes which underlie these exchanges is that people try to achieve 'a proper balance' between giving and receiving. It is clearly seen as an appropriate part of kin relationships to give and receive help. It is also apparent that this should be organised in ways which do not leave any individual in a position of net receiver, especially not in a position of overall indebtedness to another identifiable individual. It is for this reason that we have also referred to this process as keeping a proper balance between dependence and independence – it is important that no one should become 'too dependent' on someone else's assistance.

In trying to understand how people work out what 'too dependent' might mean – especially in circumstances where the exchange cannot be direct – we also need to beware of focusing too narrowly on the material value of the goods, labour or time which is being exchanged. On many occasions the negotiations seem to be less about balancing out the value of exchanges on objectively identifiable criteria, and more concerned with establishing how the nature of the exchange is to be *understood* and *treated* by the key participants. The key question often seems to be: if this gift is accepted, will it 'count' as something which unbalances the relationship significantly? What is being negotiated over is not simply – perhaps even not principally – the exchange of money, goods and labour. People are also negotiating about their position within the network of kin relationships, and the form that their specific relationships with each individual will take.

This discussion also makes it clear that issues of power and control are closely intertwined with the negotiation of the balance between dependence and independence. If a person's position gets defined as imbalanced, so that they are treated as 'too dependent' upon another relative, they end up in a position of subordination to that person. The case example of Sarah Allen's relationship with her mother brings this out very clearly. It also shows that to 'take responsibility' for helping a relative – which sounds benign and altruistic – also puts you in a position of control over that person. The basis of such control is the imbalance created by giving more to someone than they can possibly return. The nature of that power was very visible in the example of John Green's relationship with his grandchildren where he took responsibility for their financial future. This example is unusual in that John was quite comfortable about acknowledging and using the power which the imbalance in their relationship gave to him. In other examples we have tended to see this from the other side, with people worrying about the possibility of getting into a subordinate position. Many people seem keenly aware of the *potential* subordination which goes along with becoming 'too dependent' upon a relative. The English language has a phrase which expresses this well: 'I don't want to be beholden to him/her'. We have suggested that some people are more sensitively attuned to this possibility than are others, and that often it is women who are most keenly aware of it. But the idea of 'not becoming beholden' seems to be a driving force behind the way in which many people negotiate their relationships with kin.

Thus we find the concept of reciprocity useful in developing an analysis of the processes which underlie structures of support in kin groups, provided it is understood in the ways we have developed in this chapter. It is a useful beginning but it *is* only a beginning. We have left a number of ends untied in this chapter because our data raise questions which are not wholly explained by the operation of reciprocity. We would highlight three particular loose ends: the variation between one person and another in the extent to which they get locked into a pattern of reciprocal kin exchanges; that the material value of the goods and services exchanged is sometimes less important than other considerations; that power and control operate in complex ways in these exchanges, sometimes being exercised by people who apparently are in powerless positions. The concept of reciprocity is of limited value in understanding these empirical observations. The perspectives which we develop in subsequent chapters help us to take each of these further and fills out the picture which we have begun to delineate here.

3 Negotiating commitments over time

INTRODUCTION: UNDERSTANDING THE NEGOTIATION OF FAMILY RESPONSIBILITIES

Reciprocity is a process which helps considerably in understanding why and how people become committed to giving help to relatives, but it does not tell us the whole story. This was the argument of the previous chapter. In this chapter we will explore our data through a different set of analytical perspectives, in which the central concept is negotiation. We have been using the concept of negotiation as if it were unproblematic until now, but here we want to unravel what it really means in practice. It is a concept which is central to our analysis and to our argument that responsibilities between kin are not the straightforward products of rules of obligation. They are, we shall argue, the products of *negotiation*.

We need to make clear at this point what we mean by negotiation. We mean that the course of action which a person takes emerges out of his or her interaction with other people. People's behaviour cannot be explained by saying that someone is following a set of pre-ordained social rules – as for example, in the topic which we are discussing, moral rules about family responsibilities. Nor is a person's behaviour explained straightforwardly by the position which he or she occupies in the social world – for example, the idea that someone's behaviour is predetermined by the fact that she is a woman, a mother, and so on. Explanations which rely on the idea of following rules, or on the idea that action is determined by structural position in a rigid sense, leave little room for manoeuvre by individuals. By contrast the concept of negotiation emphasises that individuals do have some room for manoeuvre, though it is never entirely open-ended and sometimes it can be quite tightly constrained. In this perspective, each individual is seen as actively working out his or her own course of action, and doing so with reference to other people. It is through human interaction that people develop a common understanding of what a particular course of action will *mean*: for example, if I offer financial help to my mother in her old age, will it seem generous, or demeaning, or whatever? We are drawing here on the classic symbolic interactionist use of the concept of negotiation, and its relevance to theoretical ideas about family obligations is discussed in more detail by Finch (1989: 177–211).

Within this general definition, negotiation can take different forms. As a starting point we will make the distinction between explicit and implicit negotiations. By explicit negotiation we mean open, round-the-table discussions prompted by specific needs and events. An obvious possible occasion for explicit negotiations is when a crisis occurs in a family. A young woman has left her husband following violence, and suddenly needs somewhere to live with her children; an elderly person has a stroke and is going to need care. In such circumstances an obvious possibility is that family members consult with each other and discuss who could give what kind of help. Explicit negotiations also can occur in anticipation of situations which are likely to develop in the future, most obviously in relation to the care of an elderly person. Their essence is that they involve open discussion in which two or more parties seek to develop a common understanding of where the balance of responsibility to give and receive help should lie, in a specific set of circumstances.

Implicit negotiations contrast with this in a number of ways. What we refer to here are situations where there is no open discussion, yet people do find ways of communicating with each other about what kinds of responsibility they regard as reasonable for themselves and for other people. Such communication is likely to occur over a period of time, so that sets of commitments develop gradually, incrementally and perhaps almost unnoticed. As a consequence, when a specific need arises it seems obvious who will help.

The idea that giving help in families arises from processes of negotiation enables us to tackle some of the loose ends left at the end of the previous chapter. In particular it helps us to make sense of our empirical observation that there is wide individual variation in the extent to which people – even within the same family – get involved in helping their relatives, and acknowledge responsibilities towards them. We will argue that under-standing family responsibilities as arrived at through negotiation helps us to account for this. However we can only use the concept of negotiation to its fullest effect if we also build in the perspective of time. Negotiations about who will acknowledge what responsibilities, and towards whom, take place over long periods of time – in a sense over the whole life-time of the relevant parties. We cannot understand fully how negotiations operate without taking the long view.

Hence we use the idea of *developing commitments* as another central theme in this chapter. We argue that people become committed to accepting certain sorts of responsibilities, to particular individuals, over time. In turn this enables us to tackle another important theme which emerged in the first two chapters, and which is something of a paradox. On the one hand we have found that people do not clearly recognise or agree upon defined responsibilities attached to particular genealogical relationships. On the other hand it is clear that many people do acknowledge specific responsibilities to members of their own kin group. Our analysis in this chapter leads us to argue that a willingness to acknowledge particular sets of responsibilities emerges as commitments develop between individuals.

Because of the kind of processes which we are highlighting in this chapter we shall mainly be using our interview data, since that is where we asked people about negotiations in practice. Nevertheless, our survey data gives an indication that people publicly accept the idea of negotiations at a normative level. In Chapter 1, we noted a general tendency for there to be a stronger consensus over procedure than over the substance of family responsibilities. People are more likely to agree about factors which should be taken into account in deciding on appropriate action, than about precisely what that action should be. The very absence of a consensus over substance implies that commitments should be sorted out in other ways. In itself, this points towards an overall normative preference for negotiation about kin support. Our respondents seem to be telling us that family responsibilities should be sorted out in a process which takes various factors and contingencies into account, rather than determined on the basis of genealogical relationship or other fixed rules.

Our survey data also contain some indications that people recognise that commitments develop over time, and that this is relevant to deciding on a normatively appropriate course of action. Two of our survey vignettes specifically built a time dimension into a scenario involving personal care and practical support. Both vignettes asked at an early stage whether help should be given then, at a later stage and in the light of changing circumstances, whether it should be continued and increased. One of these vignettes, concerning Jane and Ann Hill, was discussed in detail in Chapter 2, where we saw that most people recognised the significance of the development of commitments over time between the two women. Respondents appeared to see this as an important factor which should be taken into account in deciding whether to continue the pattern of mutual aid, despite changing personal circumstances. The message is that taking on commitments means that you become more likely to attract further commitments in the future.

Our other vignette is rather different. This one concerns Jim and Margaret Robertson, and we used part of this vignette in Chapter 1 to show that people do not recognise substantive rules about *what* to do, even in parent–child relationships. The first part of the vignette was worded in this way:

> Jim and Margaret Robertson are a married couple in their early forties. Jim's parents, who live several hundred miles away, have had a serious car accident, and they need long-term daily care and help. Jim is their only son. He and his wife work for the Electricity Board and could both get tranfers so that they could work near his parents.
> What should Jim and Margaret do?
>   Move to live near Jim's parents?
>   Have Jim's parents move to live with them?
>   Give money to help pay for daily care?
>   Let them make their own arrangements?
>   Other.

The responses were concentrated in the first three options given: 33 per cent said Jim and Margaret should move, 24 per cent said Jim's parents should come to live with them, and 25 per cent said Jim and Margaret should provide money for daily care. Taken together, this represents a clear majority in favour of Jim and Margaret taking *some* responsibility (82 per cent of responses, where the consensus baseline is 37.5 per cent). However, opinion is divided on what that responsibility should involve in practice. There is certainly no consensus in favour of them becoming deeply involved in a long-term caring situation, which could be seen as the likely outcome of having Jim's parents move in with them. In the final part of the vignette, respondents were asked to consider what should be done a year later, when the circumstances had moved on:

> Jim and Margaret *do* decide to go and live near Jim's parents. A year later Jim's mother dies, and his father's condition gets worse so that he needs full-time care.
> Should Jim or Margaret give up their job to take care of Jim's father?
>   Yes, Jim should give up his job.
>   Yes, Margaret should give up her job.
>   No, neither should give up their job.
>   Don't know/depends.

Only 22 per cent said that either Jim nor Margaret should give up their jobs, and the majority view was that neither should, with 64 per cent of respondents opting for that answer (consensus baseline 50 per cent). This was the case even though respondents are given the message that Jim and Margaret have already established a commitment to Jim's parents by moving near and embarking on a personally supportive relationship with them. There is a strong message, nevertheless, that Jim and Margaret should not get further entrenched and, by implication, that they should prevent their commitment from becoming cumulative.

A comparison of the Jim and Margaret vignette with the Jane and Ann Hill one seems to suggest that people will *not* see it as normatively appropriate to continue and increase giving long-term practical support and personal care even where a commitment has been established, unless the relationship is obviously reciprocal and does not involve excessive personal cost for the carer. These messages seem less directly about the problem of imbalance between the parties, than about the danger of stepping into an apparently inexorable process of accumulating commitment. In the context of personal care then, people both recognise the force of commitments developing over time, and also want the parties to retain some control over the extent to which they accumulate.

EXPLICIT AND IMPLICIT NEGOTIATIONS IN PRACTICE

We move on now to an examination of our interview data, initially asking the questions: what evidence is there that, in practice, family responsibilities emerge from a process of negotiating? Are such negotiations implicit or explicit? We shall consider these questions by looking at our data set as a whole. We aim to give a picture of the type of help which gets negotiated, and the range of kin who negotiate with each other.

In the later part of the chapter we move directly to the question: what evidence do we have about the way commitments develop over time, and how does this part of the process work? We shall tackle that particularly complex question by means of an extended case study. While we leave the issue of developing commitments mainly to this case study, our presentation of negotiations in other examples in our data set cannot – and does not attempt to – keep the perspective of time wholly out of the picture. People's biographies, and the history of their family relationships, very clearly are brought into negotiations and shape their course.

In looking across our data set for evidence of negotiations in practice, we find that we have a large number of examples. Of itself this indicates the importance of negotiation as a significant means through which family responsibilities develop. Our examples range across the full spectrum from the totally explicit to the entirely implicit. But it becomes clear that these represent two ends of a spectrum, rather than alternative and mutually exclusive methods of negotiating. In many examples there is an element both of explicit and implicit negotiation. In presenting this range of examples we have divided them into three categories: open discussions, clear intentions, non-decisions. We should emphasise that we are not giving these categories the status of a formal typology. They are categories created to facilitate presentation and do not have watertight boundaries. Our whole point is that there is a range of ways in which people can and do negotiate with relatives, and these often contain both implicit and explicit elements.

Open discussions

Our first category is open discussions about providing support. We can identify around 136 such examples in our data set, coming from more than three-quarters of our interviewees. In these examples people told us that they or members of their family got together to discuss how to provide assistance to a relative, the appropriate division of labour between relatives and so on. The concept of a 'family conference' was used by a few people and it epitomises this form of negotiation, although not all of the interviewees were claiming that every potential family member actually got involved in discussions. In fact, we could identify no cases whatsoever where *all* relatives who were potentially affected by discussions were involved in them. Nevertheless, for our interviewees the theme – if not the reality – of 'family conference' or 'all getting together to discuss it' pervaded around half of the accounts, while the other half concerned open discussions between two or more relatives at a time. Most of the examples were first-hand accounts of negotiations which had taken place in the past. However some were third party accounts (of events which had happened elsewhere in the interviewee's kin group) and others were expectations about how particular forms of support would be arranged in the future, should the need arise. The examples include accounts of the same set of events from different members of kin groups.

Open discussions cover a wide range of types of support, and often more than one type of support was being negotiated on a single occasion. There is no straightforward relationship between the type of help being negotiated and the likelihood of open discussion, although there is a predominance of examples involving personal care of elderly or sick people (between one-third and one-half of examples involved this type of support). Various kinds of practical support were the next most likely types of support under discussion (around one-third). Financial support, and discussions about relatives providing accommodation, each emerged in around one-fifth of the examples. There were also some examples of moral support, such as generally talking things through. Negotiations were most commonly about parent–child support, although a wider range of relatives was often involved in discussions, and the full complement of parents and children were not always included.

On the surface 136 examples from over three-quarters of our interviewees is a substantial number. It suggests that open discussion is a common way in which kin responsibilities get negotiated. However, we think that conclusion could be a bit misleading for two main reasons.

First, and most importantly, the fact that people report that they talk to each other – apparently openly – about their kin responsibilities, does not automatically mean that this is the main mechanism through which kin responsibilities *get negotiated*. As we have already suggested, we are not equating negotiation with talk, but prefer to see talk – or its absence – as just one element in a more complex process of negotiation. Actually, what is important is to understand what the presence or absence of talk *means* in the context of specific negotiations. We need to look a little closer at this issue, and we will return to it shortly.

Second, and related to the question of the meaning of talk, there is a clear sense in our data that interviewees *wanted* to report open discussions; that they were rather proud of these examples. People seem actually rather pleased to be able to say that, in their family, support is negotiated openly – that they talk things through in a rational manner, to reach the best solutions. In raising this issue we are not suggesting that people's enthusiasm for the idea of family negotiations got the better of them to such an extent that they were not telling us the truth, although there may have been some 'over-reporting'. But again, it indicates that we need to examine the meaning of talk in the negotiating process, rather than taking at face value the idea that responsibilities are the straightforward products of these discussions. Jane Ashton's account of negotiations between her and her teenaged children displays some of the enthusiasm to which we are referring.

> *Jane*   It's like Christmas, we have a system that, we don't just buy anything. We'll say, 'Well what do you want', you know, like I'm having er, I have daft things at Christmas. Like I said I have clothes, our Jenny's buying me, she wanted to buy me some trousers, but I've changed my mind. So she said I can't change my mind again. I'm going to have a coat stand for the hall. You know, so that's nice. Sally's buying me, she was going to buy me a picture, I wanted a picture at first, but now I'm having new shoes.

Jane continued at length with her list of the exchange of presents between her and her children, and concluded:

> *Jane*   I mean they seem daft really, but they're useful things to me. You know what I mean, they don't go and buy loads of hankies or ladies slippers or things like that. They ask first, which I think is better. Like I'm buying our Julie a plant stand that she wants and giving Alan a voucher for a record and tape cos that's what he wants, you know. . . . But that's how we do it, that's how we go on.

In these extracts, and throughout her interviews with us, Jane is telling us that she is proud of her family, and of her relationship with her children in particular. She feels that they can and do discuss all sorts of things together, and she attributes this to having been a lone parent, and supporting them through ill-health and more than their fair share of traumatic experiences. Talk between them seems an important emblem of Jane's success as a single parent. But Jane's version of family pride is typical of many of our interviewees. Just as we argued in Chapter 2 that showing that your family 'works' at the very least means showing that relatives 'rally round' in a crisis, so the idea of being able to have discussions and negotiations is obviously attractive too. Thus we think that people were very happy to report open discussions to us, and found it easy to do so since there was something concrete to describe. By contrast, examples of more implicit forms of negotiation are more difficult to articulate. Nonetheless the large number of examples of open discussions which we have shows that these do take place quite widely, and that it is an accepted means through which definitions of family responsibilities can emerge.

Nevertheless, describing this process as 'open negotiation' makes it all sound clear-cut and simple, a straightforward way in which a family can manage 'its' affairs. However when we look below the surface this form of negotiation looks less of a purely rational process, and more complex to manage, than it first appears. In particular, these open discussions do not take place in a vacuum but within the context of a set of relationships which already exists, and will continue into the future. Also the range of possible outcomes is not totally open-ended but is limited by other considerations which are important in family life – most obviously the need to maintain the balance between dependence and independence (see Chapter 2). Essentially, when we look at an example of open discussion, what we are seeing is the tip of the iceberg.

Thus to understand the significance of an open discussion, we need to look at the content and outcome of that discussion and also at its wider context. Two connected ways of highlighting the importance of this are, first, to focus on who is excluded from discussions as well as on who is included, and second, to look at what is left unsaid as well as at what is openly discussed. We can illustrate this by looking at some examples.

A good example of this concerns three sisters, and their respective responsibilities for supporting their mother, who was becoming confused and forgetful. The account of this was given to us by Shirley Blanchflower, the daughter of one of these women. Shirley describes how her own mother, and the youngest of her mother's sisters, visit twice a week to check that their mother is alright. These two sisters have explicitly discussed the division of responsibilities. Shirley's mother does shopping while her younger sister does washing, and Shirley's father looks after the finances. All these members of the family live in the Greater Manchester region. But there is an older sister who now lives away in Cumbria, and who has not been involved in developing an agreed way of supporting their mother.

> *Shirley* There's a little bit of a bone of contention really there, because when she did live in the area for a while she got into, she went one day a week and she used to start baking her cakes and everything, so my Gran stopped baking and relied on my auntie taking stuff round. And then of course she moved away so then it left the other two to sort of carry on the situation.

What we have here is an example where responsibilities were agreed through open discussion between two sisters, but the third sister had taken a course of action without reference to them. Initially she became very involved with her mother then, following her move out of the area, excluded herself altogether. She does not seem to have discussed her position with her sisters or her mother at either stage, and apparently her sisters resent this. What is unspoken is the idea that the sister who left has broken an implicit commitment she had developed to her mother, and had been willing to discuss neither this, nor the arrangements needed to cover for the dependency she had created. Again we get the message from Shirley that open discussion is preferable in families. There is also more than a hint that one sister is denying the opportunity to the others to exert some pressure upon her to become committed to an agreed division of labour. We might surmise (though we do not have direct evidence of this) that she is adopting a 'no discussion' position in order to hold on to the initiative in her relationship with her family.

In this example the undiscussed element of the situation comes from a potential donor of help excluding herself from discussion, having been primarily responsible for cultivating the need for help in the first place. But the potential recipient can also be excluded, as the mother in this example may have been. The thinking behind such exclusion can vary, and we will consider some more examples to demonstrate this. Dorothy O'Malley had been talking to her daughter Jill about options for helping Jill's children financially as they reached adult life. The issue had been highlighted for Dorothy precisely because her eldest grand-daughter now was a young adult – so in principle she could have been involved in the discussion. But she was not. The issue had been discussed openly only by her mother and her grandmother. Jill explained it like this:

> *Jill* [My mother] wants to leave each of the children £10,000 [in her will] and she's talked about *when* to do it – what is the best age, um should

they just have it when she dies, when they die, or um should there be an age. I mean she'd thought of 30, she's thought of 20 odd. . . and, oh we haven't come to any decision about it, we don't know. She's asked me what I think and I thought, well, you know, getting a house, it would be such a leg up on your mortgage. Um [pause] when are they going to get a house? Do you do it on marriage, or do – we don't know. We're still thinking about that, I don't know.

The reasoning behind the exclusion of the recipients in a case like this can be understood in various ways. It is a major intervention in the financial affairs of a young person, and perhaps it is being treated as an issue in which older people have more experience. Alternatively, young people may be seen as needing agents or advocates to negotiate on their behalf until they are 'old enough'. Certainly, several of our 'open discussion' examples potentially affected the lives of children under 18 years old, yet in very few instances were those children actively involved in discussions. Not all of these involved financial assistance, but as we have already noted (see Chapter 2 and Appendix C), financial assistance does usually flow down the generations and excluding grandchildren from the discussion as in the O'Malley case keeps the position of recipient and donor very separate and very clear. It also preserves the control of the older generation over the exchange. Dorothy, in effect, is retaining the right to take her own decision about what she wants to do, in the light of advice from her daughter who is not a party to the transaction, in that she is not going to get anything herself from the particular pot of money being discussed.

In the O'Malley case, keeping control in the hands of the donor seems to be an important rationale for excluding the potential recipients from the discussion. We have other examples where potential recipients were excluded from discussions about support precisely so that they would not be perceived as *having had to ask* for help. Ironically, this seems more like *putting* some control in the hands of recipients because, if they had had to ask, this would have compromised their independence. Keith Pearson's negotiations with his siblings about providing their mother with a telephone helps to illustrate this.

Keith   We helped my mother out, you know with all the, we've had her a telephone put in, then she could ring any of us up if she wanted.
Interviewer   Right. What, you all sort of got together and arranged that did you?
Keith   Yes, we had to arrange it, yes.
Interviewer   Paid for it together?
Keith   Yes, we paid for it yes. We pay for her rental and all when it comes, yes, yes.

Interviewer How did that come about, did one of you decide that it was a good idea or?
Keith Er, I don't know really how it came about really. I think as she got older, we had it put in you know, and then she could er, if she ever got fed up or she were on her own, she could just ring any of us up, yes.

However, when we asked Keith further about this, it emerged that this was an idea cooked up between the siblings and then presented to their mother. Keith added that:

Keith She didn't really need us to pay for the telephone, but she *let* us do it because we kept going on about it. And then she said, it was, 'Alright, I'll let you then.' I mean she goes on holidays, she's, she's no need for any of us to support her at the moment. If she needs it, she only needs to ask and she'll get it, but er, she doesn't need it. [Emphasis in original]

In this example, the fact that Keith's mother 'let' them pay for her telephone, only after they had 'kept going on about it', illustrates the point that her exclusion from the initial discussions helped to maintain her independence because it demonstrated that she had neither asked for the support, nor even really needed it. In a sense, she is doing her children a favour by *allowing* them to give her this support: at one level, at least, she is the powerful one in this exchange.

There are other kinds of reasoning which lie behind the exclusion of certain people from open discussions. In the following case, concerning Mary Mycock's mother-in-law, the message was clearly that excluding the latter from the relevant discussion was seen as a *protection* for her. The situation was like this. The health of Mary's father-in-law had deteriorated badly, and the issue was: should he continue to be looked after at home or go into residental care? As Mary describes the situation, her husband and his siblings entered into open discussion about this and chose residental care. They deliberately excluded their mother from this discussion, on the grounds that it would be too difficult for a wife to make such a decision. Her exclusion in itself represented a significant form of support for her – they took the responsibility of the decision away from her, thus reducing her possible burden of guilt. Mary describes the situation this way:

Mary My husband was in this situation as with his mother and father and in the end the four of them, the four brothers and sisters, decided that he had to go into a hospital in, he actually went into a private hospital, private nursing home, because his mother just couldn't cope, and they, they had to take the decision off her, namely the decision he needed to go into a nursing home and it, it was a private one, it was paid for, but my mother-in [pause] my husband's mother lived till she was 93, and his father died in his early seventies.

Interviewer Oh I see, so she lived a lot longer than him?

Mary Yes, but they reckon if, if she'd carried on looking after him she'd have gone before he did because it was taking too much out of her, she just wasn't physically capable [pause] and when it's one of each it's you know husband and wife [pause] if the children don't live close enough they just can't give enough support, and it's 24 hours a day and it's too much.

Interviewer It's interesting that in that case the children all got together and talked about it, did they, and decided that that was . . . ?

Mary They made the decision. Because she wouldn't make the decision – well she can't, you can't expect a husband and wife to make that sort of decision. It has to be taken out of their hands, I'd say, you know.

There is an analytical distinction between exclusions which are intended to protect people, or to maintain an appropriate level of independence (by removing the *need* for someone to participate in discussions, or to have to ask for help), and those which are intended to disempower (by removing the *right* to participate). However, the latter may sometimes become the unintended consequence of the former, and in any case the interpretations of the different parties to the same set of negotiatons may diverge on this matter.

In considering our 'open discussions' category we have concentrated on explaining the undiscussed elements in the negotiations which lie below the 'tip of the iceberg'. In particular, we have examined the exclusion of certain relevant individuals. We have seen that such exclusions can be quite deliberate – whether exclusion of oneself or of other people. But being deliberate does not necessarily mean that there is a malicious intent – indeed it can be quite the reverse. In some examples such exclusions seem to be a conscious strategy, in others it is much less clear that they are the result of strategic thinking of that sort.

Thus looking at who is excluded, on what basis, and what is left unsaid, helps us to fill out our understanding of what is happening in these open discussions. We find in our examples of open discussions that explicit negotiations are a well-established feature of family life, indeed that they are valued as a sign of strong family relationships, but that there is a lot more going on. This helps us to understand something about how family responsibilities develop provided it is treated cautiously, we have argued. However, this is by no means the only way in which kin negotiate with each other about giving and receiving help.

Clear intentions

We have characterised our second category of methods of negotiating as 'clear intentions'. These are examples where people have consciously planned how to provide support, and sometimes implicitly got that message over to other people involved, without actually bringing it out into the open for discussion. We have around forty-five examples in our data set of clear intentions which apparently did not involve any open discussion. Again they cover a wide range of support, including practical (12), accommodation (15), financial (12) personal care (12), household organisation (3). The support being negotiated over was concentrated in the parent–child range (16 parent–child where the support was to be provided up the generations; 7 parent–child down the generations; 11 where direction was not clear or was being established through negotiations; 11 other genealogical relationships).

If someone has formed a clear intention to give help, why is there no open discussion? In some instances the reason for not speaking openly about it was fairly clear, in others it was not. Where the reason was clear, often it was similar to the logic governing the exclusion of certain people from open discussions: that is, it was concerned with maintaining the dependence–independence balance. Open discussion of the issue would, it seems, disturb this more than the actual giving and receiving of help. For example, in the following case, Sarah Yates talks about the help which her mother has given to her in recent years, by doing the washing and ironing for Sarah's household every week. This is valuable practical assistance for Sarah but it also represents emotional support for her mother, giving her a way of adjusting to her widowhood. However, Sarah's mother has recently become ill, and Sarah is now facing a dilemma.

> *Sarah* She's developed angina. So now I'm going to have to be very careful what I do with her, because (a) I don't want her to think that she's an invalid because that'll make her worse, er a lot of people her age get angina, it's not unusual, and (b) I've got to cut the washing down or how she does it, down, um its been a bit heavy for the last six weeks because with the school being off, my daughter tends to change her clothes three times a day [laughs], which of course now she's realised is not so good, she's prepared to not wear as many clothes, but basically I've got to cut her down on some of either the washing or the ironing and, but without her being hurt.

Sarah is saying that she has a clear intention to reduce the amount of help which her mother gives her, but that to do so openly could compromise the delicate balance of dependence and independence in their relationship. The reasons for keeping quiet about a clearly formulated intention are easy to see in this case, once one listens carefully to what is being said. Similar reasoning is reflected in a number of other cases in our data set, though sometimes not as clearly as it is here. It seems quite commonly to be a way in which parents and children in particular manage their relationship, at different points in their lives.

The dependence–independence balance was not the sole factor lying behind cases where clear intentions were left publicly unstated, however. In some cases the unspoken nature of the transaction seemed to be more a way of ensuring that the potential recipient of help was not put in a position where she or he had to ask for it, just as the exclusion of people – like Keith Pearson's mother – from open discussions could be interpreted in a similar way. An example of this was given to us by Jean Crabtree, and concerned a time several years previously when she had been a young, single woman living with her widowed mother.

> *Jean* Well, up until when my grandma got very ill, er she [mother] had always sort of made the tea for me, done my washing, that type of thing, er but once she started to look after my grandma more, what happened was I used to er, do shopping for myself and get, buy my own food, instead of giving her housekeeping money for food, I used to buy my own food and do my own cooking for myself, and just give her money for things like the, you know, towards the house, electricity and the phone, that type of thing. So I would do my own washing and ironing, so I became more independent then, because I was trying to help her, knowing that she had so much work to do, you know, helping my grandma and grandad [pause] I had to try and do something, so that was my way, you know, of helping her.

The essence of Jean's consideration here seems to have been to seize the initiative, and to ensure that her mother was not embarrassed by having to solicit her daughter's help. The phenomenon of 'not having to ask' is an important one in transactions between kin, and we explore it directly in Chapter 5.

Some other examples of 'clear intentions' also emphasise seizing the initiative, but in a different way. There are a few cases where discussion was not entered into because the donor wanted no dispute about what was to be done. By formulating a clear intention, then simply acting on it, this person is stating that there *should* be no discussion. An example of this comes from our interview with Avril King, a middle-aged woman who had nursed her mother through a terminal illness several years previously, with little help from her two brothers. In the following extract Avril describes how her mother started giving her gifts of various household items.

> *Avril* Funnily enough, my mother had started to give me things, now my

mother must have known she was ill [pause]. Er, well those days they didn't have duvets, they had you know the candlewick, such gorgeous bedding, she kept giving me these. Not even out of the packets, er, you know, Avril she said 'Take that' I said 'No mum, I don't want it' 'I want *you* to have it now.' My mum made sure I did get some things, she kept giving me things over a period of time, and I think she knew, that um, she was ill, and er I mean when I think back. [Emphasis in original]

In this extract Avril's mother is acting in a way which brooks no dissent. If she had initiated open discussions, she would effectively have been disempowering herself. She wants Avril specifically to get these items ('I want *you* to have it') and in the circumstances Avril was in no position to debate this. Significantly, the other people also unable to debate this as a consequence were Avril's brothers, and the full meaning of their mother's actions becomes clear elsewhere in Avril's interview. After her mother died, her brothers had the pick of her belongings, Avril told us, despite the fact that they had contributed little to her care. What she is telling us in the extract above is that her mother anticipated this possibility and took action to ensure that Avril got a fair share. Open discussions may well have precluded that possibility.

Thus this particular style of negotiating family obligations – formulating clear intentions but not putting them up for open discussion – can occur for a variety of reasons. In most cases the desire to avoid discussion seems strategic, for reasons which are comprehensible when we know enough about the relationships involved. In that sense, formulating clear intentions should be considered part of the process of negotiating family obligations, though implicit rather than explicit.

Non-decisions

Our final category of types of negotiation is entitled 'non-decisions'. By this we mean the process of reaching an understanding about family responsibilities without *either* open discussion *or* any party having formed a clear intention, in so far as we can tell. We include this category for completeness, as it represents the end of the spectrum where negotiations are most implicit. However, there is a sense in which many of the examples which we use in other chapters also illustrate non-decisions. In very many cases when people talk about how they (or someone else) came to accept responsibility for helping a particular relative, they cannot reconstruct a consciously formulated strategy, or identify a point in time when there was an overt agreement. The arrangement just emerged. It became obvious that a certain person would help. In the same way, many of the examples of 'clear intention' or 'open discussion' from this chapter have elements of non-decisions within them. For example, sometimes – even when there was open discussion about how support should be provided – the decision about who should provide support had already 'been taken' implicitly, or had become obvious over time. These are the themes which we encounter over and over again in our interviews.

Nevertheless, we have been able to separate out a group of examples which we might call 'clear non-decisions', where people told us that definitely there was no discussion, that help was just given – or in a few cases, that this is how matters will be conducted in their families in the future. Forty-six of our interviewees (i.e. just over half) gave us at least one example of this kind. There may well be many more cases not reported to us in this way, because implicit processes tend to be more difficult to identify and recount than more concrete examples of open discussion.

A minority of cases in the non-decisions category seemed to be examples of people making a statement about their families by reference to the meaning of talk – and in this case its absence – in the negotiating process. While some people may take pride in claiming that theirs is a family which uses open discussion, rather ironically others may be proud of not *having to* have discussions. We do not think this is contradictory, because in a sense both versions involve taking pride in the same thing: that your family 'works' in the sense that everyone rallies round in a crisis (see Chapter 2 where this idea is first developed). One way of saying that may be to report that members of your family discuss things openly; another may be to say that rallying round takes place automatically, without discussion.

A typical example of pride in non-decision-making to illustrate these points comes from the Jackson kin group. The following extract is from Robert Jackson's interview, where he gives a good example of a non-decision – in this case anticipating a situation which may occur in the future. He has been talking about his father's ill-health, and goes on to consider what he and his two brothers will do if his mother is widowed.

Robert   Eventually, not looking too far in the future, there's going to be a lot of responsibility that we've got to, the three of us have got to undertake.
Interviewer   Have you discussed it between the three of you?
Robert   No.
Interviewer   You've not, it hasn't been discussed, no.
Robert   No, it's something that doesn't need discussing. We all know that eventually it's going to happen and we all know what each is, what each is going to do.
Interviewer   What, that one will do one sort of thing, and one will do another, sort of?

Robert Well you see, *again* because I've been a policeman, all the funeral side is down to me, because I'm hard. They always say 'Oh you're hard to it anyway.' So when it comes down to arrangements and so on and so forth, I know exactly what has to be done, so they won't even consider doing anything like that. Er, my first eldest'll [brother] look after my mother, because he's the one round the corner, so he'll be there all the time. The other one will deal with all the relations, all the relatives that need to know. He'll deal with that side. We don't even need to talk about it, because we know that that's how it's going to happen. It's a strange inbuilt feeling that we've all got you know. [Emphasis in original]

In his account, Robert rejects the whole idea of open discussion about family responsibilities, and indicates that his family would proceed by non-decision-making. We see Robert's account as a version of the theme of 'not having to ask' for help. The message he seems to be trying to convey is that he and his brothers will not wait to be asked by anyone to help, but will come forward and offer their contributions. As a way of demonstrating this, he tells us that they already know – without need for discussion – what those contributions will be. Whether or not this implicitly agreed division of labour would *actually* be activated without discussion is not certain, however. On the face of it our interview with one of Robert's brothers, McNeil, gives a different impression. McNeil does not share his brother's clear view of what their division of labour in this situation would be. He says he does not know what they would do, and certainly does not give the impression that they have implicitly worked this out between them. Not least this is because he has not wanted to anticipate his father's death, even implicitly. However, although McNeil's account diverges from Robert's in that he feels that discussion *would* be necessary to work out what to do, the message they both make very clear is that they would want to do all they could, and would not wait to be asked to make a contribution. Both brothers share the view that theirs is a family that rallies round in a crisis.

In this sense, pride in non-decision-making may not be that different from pride in being able to discuss things openly: both may be versions of the message that your family works, in the sense that everybody pulls together when needed.

However, most of the examples of non-decisions involve only one or two people taking responsibility, rather than a group effort as is suggested in the Jackson case. In these cases, there is one striking way in which our non-decisions category differs from the other two categories. Here we find that the focus is principally on women, as the 'obvious' people to take responsibility. Examples where there has been (or will be) no discussion have a strong gendered dimension. The end result is most likely to be that *a woman* accepts responsibility for providing assistance. By contrast, examples of open discussion may result in either women or men taking responsibility. As it happens, many of our examples of non-decisions are about personal care, where the outcome is that a woman accepts responsibility. Our qualitative data set as a whole does show a preponderance of women over men providing personal care (around twice as many, as documented in Appendix C), and it seems significant that they are concentrated in this non-decisions category. By contrast, very few men end up accepting responsibility for personal care through a process of non-decisions. Where men provide such care, their responsibilities have usually been negotiated through open discussions with other people.

Let us consider some examples to illustrate these points. Some were given by women who seemed to regret that their own responsibilities were obvious to everyone. Avril King provides an example of this:

Avril At home, you see, I've got two older brothers, you see I'm the baby, and my mother took ill of cancer [pause] and um [pause] I mean I was the one, um, that you know, did everything. I mean I was working full-time at that particular time, I had a very responsible job, but I had a very good boss, who said you know, if I ever needed to, to go home, I could. But um, you see, that all fell on me. I mean the lads didn't do much at all really.
Interviewer Was that because you were living nearby?
Avril Well I was here. Again, you see, they were just down the road and um, but they, they're, I mean, not miles away [laughs] you know what I mean. They're only in a place called Offerton which isn't, by car, is ten minutes, you know, my elder brother doesn't, they don't have a car, but my other one does and, um, but there again, that fell on me.
Interviewer Do you think that was, to do with, because you were the daughter, or not?
Avril Don't know really, but my sister-in-law, they never really bothered [pause] you know, they never er, I mean. When Miles's [Avril's husband] mother was only 58 we found her dead in bed and um, I mean, right away, you know 'you come to our house for Sunday dinner, you do . . .'. 'Well he [Miles's father] was working shifts at the time. 'I'll do all your washing and ironing.' It was automatic for me to do that, you know. But my sister-in-laws, they never even came to see if they could help in any way when my mum was ill [pause] you know. It was, I mean I've got a very good husband, you know, who was very good [pause] and er, but it all fell on me.

When Avril is asked whether she seemed the obvious person because of her gender, she tells the story of her involvement with her husband's parents as a daughter-in-law, and reflects that her mother's daughters-in-law did not show a similar commitment. She clearly does not think that gender is a straightforward explanation. But whatever the explanation, we get a picture of Avril stepping in to help without discussion, and other people assuming that she would, or taking for granted that she did.

Another example concerned a woman whom we did not interview, but about whom we have several accounts from members of the Jones kin group (see Appendix A for kin group details): from her sister, from her niece and from her grand-niece. This woman perhaps fitted the classic stereotype of the spinster-carer: she had lived with her parents until their death, and had been involved not only in their care, but in the care of several other relatives both before and after her parents' death. The accounts we have from her sister, her niece and her grand-niece, all emphasise the extent to which everyone viewed her as the obvious family carer. Her sister, Kathleen Snow, explains the situation like this:

> *Interviewer* Do you think it's because of the type of person she is that she's got involved like this, or because she was living, was sort of handy, or . . . ?
>
> *Kathleen* Well, I think circumstances *make* you what you *are* don't they, because if she hadn't had all these old people, if she had got married when she was younger, and gone to live away, this probably would never have cropped up. It just happens that where you are at a certain time, doesn't it?
>
> *Interviewer* Yes, yes. Was she working, did she have a job?
>
> *Kathleen* No she wasn't working no, she had worked when she was younger, but she wasn't working then.

And finally, one of the rare examples where a man was seen at least by some relatives as obvious carer. This example concerns the brother of one of our interviewees, Eileen Simpson. Eileen has three brothers. Two are married with children, and the other, in his fifties, is single, and lives with Eileen's 80-year-old widowed father who is still fairly fit and active. Her brother has effectively never moved away from home, and is now increasingly involved in looking after their father. In our interviews with Eileen's husband, and two of their young adult children, we get the idea that the supportive relationship between her brother and father has evolved fairly naturally, as a result of non-decisions 'taken' over time. Eileen's perception although similar in theme, is slightly different.

> *Eileen* He [father] lives over in Birmingham, my brother lives with him. My brother didn't marry. I feel guilty about my brother more than I do my father actually, funnily enough, because I feel he has [pause] all

the problems of it [pause] although my father at the moment is still quite fit, he can still get out and about – he's 80 in April – but he still needs looking after if you like. He doesn't get meals or anything like that so that falls on my brother. And keeping the house clean and everything falls on my brother, although they've got a home help for two hours once a week. I mean what that does I mean is nothing really. Um, since we've been working in the shop I feel guilty because I haven't been able to get over there. I used to go over, because I've got the car, once a week at least just to see how he was going, but there was *nothing I could do*. This is what I felt useless at, because my brother, he's very capable. I mean he always kept the house clean. My father would never let me cook him a meal. He'd always want a sandwich. [Emphasis in original]

In this example we do get a sense of the implicit negotiations and indeed struggles that can go on around non-decisions. Eileen has not been particularly comfortable with the idea that her brother is the obvious and natural carer for their father.

Taken together, we think these data suggest that different negotiating processes may apply to women and men, especially around the issues of caring. These processes need to be understood as tied into women's and men's biographies and the different ways in which these usually get woven into commitments which develop over time. By this reckoning, Eileen Simpson's brother was 'selected' through a non-decision-making process because of an unusual (for men) biography, which provided the conditions for the development of commitment between him and his father specifically. As a result, he came to be in a position where he could be seen as an obvious carer, without discussion. The point really is that it is usually women's biographies which put them in a position where they can be regarded as an obvious carer without the need for discussion. Men's biographies do not, except unusually.

This example demonstrates that the process of negotiation can only be understood with reference to the biographies of the individuals involved and the history of their relationships, as they have developed over time. Biographies themselves are part of the negotiating process. Assumptions about who will do what for whom, and in what way, are built upon previous negotiations and the reputations people have established through their conduct in those negotiations. Outcomes get carried forward and expressed in continuing biographies, and in developing commitments. As we have argued above, these also tend to inform the more explicit forms of negotiation. We have no cases where the pattern and division of responsibility emerged entirely out of discussions in a vacuum. However, that does not mean that the outcomes of negotiations are predetermined.

FORMS OF NEGOTIATING PRACTICE

Our aim in this section has been to demonstrate the importance of negotiation as a mechanism through which family responsibilities emerge. The large number of examples in our data set underlines this. All types of practical and financial assistance get negotiated in families. Any relevant relatives may be involved. Though in the majority of our examples parents and children predominate, this reflects our range of examples of kin support more generally (see Appendix C) rather than telling us anything specifically about negotiations. The preponderance of negotiations in the parent–child range does, however, add weight to our argument that family responsibilities are not the products of substantive rules pertaining to genealogical relationships, even for parents and children. If there were clear rules about what parents and children should do for each other, we would expect to see many fewer examples of negotiation in practice.

Through discussion of examples of negotiation in three different categories, we have tried to show the wide range of approaches which people take to the business of negotiating family responsibilities. Both explicit and implicit mechanisms are used widely, often together.

In general our interviewees endorse the virtue of open discussion in families. Being able to discuss such matters openly, to arrive at an agreed division of labour, is a sign that a family is working well in most people's eyes. It shows that everyone is prepared to acknowledge responsibilities and to pull their weight (see Chapter 2, and also Finch and Mason, 1990b; 1991). If everyone pulling their weight in the division of responsibilities is ideally what a family should express, then open discussion is a mechanism through which this outcome can be seen to be achieved. Thus people were pleased if they were able to report that open discussions did take place, and conversely could show displeasure with a particular relative who did not take part in them.

Interestingly, however, the logic of all this can work the other way round. In a few cases, people were actually proud of the fact that their family did *not* talk openly about who should do what. In these cases, the logic seems to be that 'we do not *have to*' discuss what is going to happen – people just get on and do it. In contrast with the other examples, in these cases not having to discuss was taken as a sign that the family was working well, in the sense that people all pulled their weight automatically. Nevertheless, we do not think this indicates that people were operating with kinship rules about who should do what, which made either discussion or negotiation unnecessary. Instead, we interpret this as a version of the theme of 'not having to ask, or be asked'.

In a sense, in our non-decisions and open discussions categories we seem to be picking up on two different versions of a theme we mentioned in Chapter 2, that rallying round in a crisis is a way of showing that your family 'works'. For many people, rallying round means showing that you are prepared to have a family conference and sort out what to do. For others, though, it means showing that you will all come forward with offers of help, rather than waiting to be asked.

We have also highlighted the importance of looking at what is not discussed openly, and who is not included in explicit negotiations. Refusal to enter discussion, or the exclusion of someone else from open discussion, emerge as important phenomena in the negotiating process. These mechanisms are not necessarily a way simply of avoiding taking on responsibilities. Often they are quite the reverse – an integral part of the process of giving help can be that it is not openly discussed. Given the fact that, in general, open discussion is valued highly this may seem rather curious. But exclusion of oneself or someone else from open discussion becomes entirely understandable when one knows enough about the context, and often seems to be a way of managing the relationships of power and control inherent in these negotiations. Most clearly, we have been able to show that staying out of open discussion enables a person to retain more control over the situation, which may be very important if they are someone who might give assistance to a relative. Staying out of open discussion enables more control to remain in the hands of the donor. In entering open discussion about a divison of labour between relatives, one inevitably is relinquishing such control – though obviously others also may be in the same position. The importance of ensuring that power remains in the hands of the donor is a theme which we take up directly in Chapter 5.

In general therefore, our interview data support the view that negotiation is a widespread phenomenon in relation to family responsibilities, and that mechanisms for negotiation can take a variety of different forms. But precisely how it all works, and especially how it develops over time, is something which can only be fully understood by looking at the process in greater detail. We move therefore to consideration of a single case, in order to tease out these elements more effectively.

NEGOTIATING COMMITMENTS IN PRACTICE: A CASE STUDY

For this case we have selected the Simpson kin group, where we are capitalising on having interviewed several members of the family. It is particularly useful to present data in this way on the topic of negotiation because it enables us to build up a picture of how the commitments which were developing appeared to different parties.

We have chosen the Simpson family, not because their experiences are particularly typical or atypical, but because their relationships display all the processes which we are trying to understand. They give us examples of negotiations which have explicit as well as implicit elements, and also of processes of gradually accumulating commitments. We are not going to attempt to discuss all the rich data which we have on this family. We are confining ourselves to negotiations and renegotiations about the position of one member of the family, Doreen (the grandmother), and how other people's commitments to her developed over time. Some of the material we use in this case study is of a sensitive nature, so we have used substitute pseudonyms, and have changed certain details which do not affect the analysis.

We interviewed four members of the Simpson family: Julie, her father Stan, her mother Eileen and her sister Janet. Julie was interviewed first in our survey, and then again twice in our qualitative study. Because she was our key interviewee, the kin group is 'hers', in the sense that it is constructed around those people she counted as her immediate family. At the time of our qualitative interviews, Julie was 25 years old, single and lived alone in her own flat in Manchester. She was a graduate, and was working full-time as a computer programmer.

One of Julie's sisters, Janet, was our second interviewee. She was 21 years old, single and lived alone in a rented flat near Leeds, a couple of miles from their parents. She worked full-time as an insurance clerk, and unlike Julie had not been to university. Stan and Eileen Simpson, their parents, were our third and fourth interviewees. Aged 52 and 46 years respectively, they lived in their own house in Leeds. Stan had worked for the same company for over twenty years, originally in sales, and latterly in management. In 1986 he was made redundant, and since then he and Eileen have been running a grocery shop. Eileen's employment career has been less continuous and was broken for childbearing and rearing. She has worked in a variety of jobs – technical, clerical and shop work. Running the grocery shop is the first full-time job Eileen has had for many years.

We were unable to interview two other members of Julie's 'immediate' kin group: her grandmother, Doreen, and her sister, Clare. Doreen is Stan's 80-year-old mother. She has been living with Eileen and Stan since shortly after she was widowed some eighteen years ago, and the household has moved twice during that time. She has not been employed for many years. Clare is one year younger than Julie. She is divorced and living with her new partner in Essex. She works full-time, and like Janet has not had a university education.

The initial issue: how to respond to Doreen's widowhood?

We enter the lives of this family when, some eighteen years ago, Stan and Eileen Simpson offered Doreen Simpson a home with them. At the time Doreen was in her sixties and had recently been widowed. On the face of it, there is no obvious reason why this particular course of action should have been chosen, or why it was Stan and Eileen who initiated it. First of all, Doreen was – and still is – fit and well. She did not need personal care of the round-the-clock kind which might have prompted Stan and Eileen to feel they needed to be in the same household as her. Second, the arrangement was intended from the start to be a permanent one. It cannot be explained as a temporary measure to give Doreen time to sort herself out after the death of her husband. And third, Doreen had another son and a daughter, both married, living no more than an hour's journey away.

So the particular circumstances of this case do not immediately suggest a reason for Stan and Eileen's offering Doreen a home. Also this would not have been seen as an 'obvious' move in the more general sense of its being a common response to widowhood. In the white British community at least, rather few elderly people live with their children – no more than 5 per cent according to national data (Arber et al., 1988; Wall, 1989). Our own interview data reflect this position. Appendix C shows that we had only four examples of elderly people living with their children on a permanent basis at the time we conducted the interviews, of whom two in fact were in households of Asian descent. In three of these four cases, the adult child had always shared a home with their parent, bringing their own spouse into this arrangement, rather than setting up the co-residence after a period living in separate households. The fourth case is the Simpsons.

On the face of it, therefore, the Simpsons' course of action is quite puzzling. Why was Doreen offered a permanent home after being widowed, and why did this offer come from Stan and Eileen rather than anyone else? In order to understand this, we need to look at the process of negotiation which went on around the time that the offer was made, and at the way in which that process was rooted in a set of relationships which had their own ongoing dynamics.

The four members of the Simpson family whom we interviewed all gave remarkably similar versions of the reasoning behind the offer, and all of their accounts depend for their logic on the assumption that Stan in particular had *already* developed a strong sense of personal responsibility for Doreen and her well-being, prior to her widowhood. The sudden death of her husband from a heart attack, however, changed the nature of her needs, and the question for Stan was how best could he *continue* to support her. Eileen explains their reasoning in the following way:

Eileen   Stan has always been very very fond of his mother, both his parents, and certainly he was close to his mother, and she was on her own at that time and he was worried about her. Also the fact, it was not all one-sided. It was a little bit selfish on our part as well because she'd got a big garden, that house. He was also picking her up every weekend after his father died and bringing her over to us, which was a bit of a bind. He used to pick her up on Friday evening and then take her back on the Sunday evening, which tied every weekend we had. You know, we hadn't got any freedom if you like, but we felt she shouldn't be on her own for too long. Then also it was the fact of keeping the house up if there were any jobs wanted to be done. You know, that's a problem, the gardening. So we thought about it and we, we got on well and we decided if she *would*, it would be better for her to come to us than for him to have that, you know, and she was only 60 at the time so, as you know, it could have gone on for years.

Eileen's main concern at this stage was Stan's well-being, rather than anxiety about Doreen specifically. Stan already felt committed: it was not an option to reduce his visiting time and practical support for Doreen. The issue for them both became how to make it all manageable. Under these circumstances the particular solution of sharing a household makes much more sense. However, both Eileen and Stan knew that making this offer would have implications for Eileen. It would draw her into a more direct involvement with Doreen than she had experienced previously. Stan alludes to this when he says:

Stan   I was the one mother turned to [pause] and because in particular Eileen and mother got on so well, um we eventually made the decision that she come and live with us.

Stan knew he was beginning to involve Eileen actively in responsibility for his mother, and needed her approval for doing that. The explicit element of their negotiation focused around this, where both could anticipate a change in the pattern of their relationships as a consequence of making their offer to Doreen. Initially Stan and Eileen just discussed it together, drawing no one else in. Like other examples given earlier they were excluding other relevant parties from the discussion at this stage, and retaining control over it themselves until they were ready to go more public. The process they both describe is one of a reasoned, round-the-table discussion, exploring options, agreeing what they would be prepared to do. Only once that process had been finalised did they draw Doreen in, by offering her a permanent home: an offer which they were by no means certain she would accept but, as Stan put it, 'We thought it was right that it should come from us.' There is more than a trace of searching for an appropriate balance between dependence and independence here (see Chapter 2); of not putting Doreen in a position where she had to *ask* for more support, and of presenting the deal as one whereby all involved would benefit. Like many of the respondents in our survey (see Chapter 1) they were as much concerned with the procedural aspects of the negotiations (how they were conducted) as with their substance (what the outcome would be).

These procedural aspects of the negotiations have had lasting implications, as Stan implies when he says, 'We asked her to come, which she reminds v~ of on occasions [laughs]. We did ask her to come and live with us.' Dore has evidently reminded Stan and Eileen on occasion that they bear the re onsibility for offering her a home. Eileen's comments imply that this wa nade clear in negotiations at the outset: 'She did want to come although she d advise us they were long livers in their family and, you know, to think a ut it.'

A similar process reflected in the involvement in the negotiations of Stan's siblings. Stan Eileen informed the siblings of the offer they intended to make, prior approaching Doreen. They had not expected the siblings to make a similar er, since they already had less sustained contact with Doreen, and had no veloped such a strong commitment to her. Therefore the siblings were involved in the negotiations about *what* to do, but were asked to respond what Stan and Eileen *proposed* to do. Their reactions were different: Stan ister advised that Stan and Eileen should proceed with caution, saying 's and think, don't jump in or you might regret it'. His brother, on the o hand, 'thought it was a great idea'. Although different, both reactio effectively re-emphasised Stan and Eileen's responsibility for their o r, rather than challenging it. Our interviewees did not actually use the p se 'you've made your bed, you lie on it', but that seems to conjure up t recautionary message about the future which was being conveyed.

At this stage the significance of th utcomes of negotiations was therefore twofold. First, the decision taken would almost inevitably create an unequal provision of material goods and services between Stan, Eileen and Doreen on the one hand, and Doreen and her other children on the other hand. Second, the division of responsibility was underlined symbolically. Everybody knew what it meant. The *meaning* of the help offered was being negotiated as well as the form it would take. There was more at stake here than material issues concerning who did what for whom. What was also taking place was the entrenching of *moral* commitments and responsibilities within the kin group.

The continuing issue: developing commitments in the Simpson family

Thus a pattern of commitments began to develop through the explicit negotiations about sharing a household. Obviously this pattern was not entirely new. Those negotiations were not conducted in a vacuum, but in the context of pre-existing relationships and commitments which had developed over time. Stan already felt a stronger responsibility to Doreen than did his siblings, and his offer of a home was partly made because he felt that, whatever needed to be done, it would be he and not his siblings that would do it. During the eighteen years since that time, this pattern has been consolidated. In a sense, we would expect that, given existing research which demonstrates that people who provide within-household care and support tend to become more, not less, responsible for continuing to do so (Qureshi and Walker, 1989). But in the Simpsons' case, we can trace the actual processes through which this has happened. There are four distinct strands.

First of all, over the years Doreen, Stan and Eileen have got involved in everyday exchanges of practical support, which have helped to strengthen the commitments between them, in comparison with the commitments between Doreen and her other children. The opportunity to give and receive help of all types was enhanced once Doreen was living in the household. The dynamics of reciprocity have ensured a process of consolidation. Stan put it like this:

> *Stan*   It's not just been one way, even now, my mother's in her eightieth year, and in the last five weeks Eileen and I would hardly have had a cooked meal if it hadn't been for my mother. She's been here so, and Eileen's very appreciative of that, you know [laughs]. And when we've had illness like, thankfully not very often but, if its been Eileen then there's been mother and myself to look after her as well as the girls. And a few times my mother's been ill and we haven't had to go trekking backwards and forwards, she's been here and we've been able to look after her. OK it's fallen mainly on Eileen because I've been working.

As a result of sharing a household, Eileen in particular began to take on a greater personal commitment to Doreen than she had previously. In Stan's words, 'it's fallen mainly on Eileen', and in a sense we can see that the conditions were right for a commitment to develop between the two women: Eileen was initially at home looking after her children, and in later years employed part-time, so she was there with Doreen more than Stan could be because of his job. What is more, the types of help Doreen could contribute, and also the support she needed, were mainly of a domestic nature, and that meant negotiations with Eileen who held the primary responsibility for the domestic sphere. Therefore although the division of responsibility between

Stan and Eileen on the one hand, and his siblings on the other, has been consolidated, there has been a gradual and incremental change in the division *between Stan and Eileen* from the days when Stan was travelling to his mother's house to give her practical help. But, if Eileen's more direct responsibility for helping Doreen has developed gradually, it was not entirely unanticipated at the outset. Stan's precondition for sharing a household – that his mother and his wife could get on well together – suggests that this was an implicit part of the bargain.

Second, the process of consolidation has had explicit as well as implicit elements. All of our interviewees talked about one event which occurred some ten years after Doreen had been sharing a household with the Simpsons, which clearly they all saw as significant in the way relationships developed. Basically this was an argument within the household about the use of space and living rooms. Although Doreen had her own bedroom, up until then she had shared living space with the rest of the family. The conflict was resolved by marking out a living room for Doreen's personal use. The importance of this event for the division of responsibilities lies less in its content, however, than in the way the siblings were drawn in. Eileen alludes to this when she says, 'We did have, er, a flare up, and she was going to leave. But of course no one wanted her, which was very hurtful for her obviously.' In fact, during the conflict, Doreen said she would go and live with one of her other children, but when this was put to them they rejected the idea. This very clearly underscored the existing division of responsibility in two ways: in material terms it eliminated one potential alternative arrangement, and in moral terms it helped to establish that, as Eileen put it later, the siblings 'are not above refusing'.

It is apparent from this series of events that the process of developing commitments between Stan, Eileen and Doreen continued to affect other people, and other people's actions continued to affect the course of the developing relationship between these three. This is the third strand which we can identify in the process of developing commitments in the Simpson case – the web of relationships within the kin group. The way in which other people positioned themselves constrained the options available to Stan, Eileen and Doreen. Conversely their actions affected the options open to others. This process is clearest in relation to the role of Stan's siblings, to which we have already referred. The fact that Stan and Eileen had taken overall responsibility created conditions which were not conducive to the siblings strengthening their commitments to Doreen. Partly, this is because, as Stan puts it, 'Over the years I think we felt they'd taken us for granted because mother lived with us.'

Certainly, if the siblings were to stop helping altogether, it seems likely that Stan and Eileen would carry on, but if the situation were reversed so that

Stan and Eileen were to stop, the siblings have already made it clear that they would not take over. Janet, the youngest daughter, explains the difference in their positions in the following way:

> *Janet*   My parents have always said they wouldn't put my grandmother into a home, there's no way because they wouldn't want to be put into a home when they got older. So I mean by saying that, that means they are putting it on to themselves because, it sounds horrible, but I'm pretty sure the other two would say 'Well she will have to go into a home' and that's it. But my mum and dad won't allow it, but *because* they won't allow it the other two are likely to turn round and say 'Well if you won't allow it, you'll have to take the responsibility of it.' [Emphasis in original]

Janet is talking about the future, and what would be done in the event that Doreen began to need personal care. But there is already evidence that the siblings do not feel a responsibility to share commitments which flow from Stan and Eileen's decision to offer Doreen a home. For example, all of our Simpson interviewees felt that the siblings had not helped Stan and Eileen enough over the years, and particularly that they had not done enough to give them some 'privacy'. Julie puts it like this:

> *Julie*   Mum and Dad have a lot more to bear than the others do and I don't think they really pull their weight. There's lots of things, little things like the odd weekend saying 'Come over to us for Sunday' or something which they don't do and they could and it really wouldn't upset them so much. Whereas it would give Mum and Dad and break. Some privacy really. Because that's the main thing, I mean they just do not have the house to themselves very often and they should have that.

Julie is saying that her aunt and uncle, in her view, have an obligation to help *her parents* because they have taken total responsibility for Doreen and as a result do not get any free time. However, the help that her parents need is directly related to the particular way in which they chose to give support to Doreen. This is the key factor which makes the siblings much less likely to see it as their responsibility to help; the needs flow from a decision about helping Doreen which was not theirs.

Thus the conditions created by Stan and Eileen's initial actions, when they accepted the overall responsibility for Doreen's welfare, militate against any further strengthening of Stan's siblings' commitment to her. They have, in short, set a course where Doreen's relationships with all her children were bound to be altered, and theirs with each other. These conditions also have had an interesting effect upon the relationship between Stan and Eileen and their own daughters. As the situation has developed, Janet in particular has been drawn into helping ease the burdens connected with supporting her grandmother. She sees this explicitly as giving help to *her parents*, her mother in particular, rather than to her grandmother. She is helping them to carry their responsibility – the same logic that Julie had used when she said that her aunt and uncle should be helping her parents, rather than that they should be helping her grandmother. Janet explains her involvement like this:

> *Janet* I took my grandmother shopping on Monday to get her Christmas shopping because it was going to fall on my mum and with her working full-time, they're very busy in the shop trying to get things organised and learning a lot of things, and my Mum just doesn't get enough time at the moment to do her own housework, or she doesn't know when she's going to get her own Christmas shopping done. And both my auntie and my uncle have made it quite clear that they couldn't possibly take my grandmother shopping so I took her shopping in the end. It *annoyed* me in a little way that I had to do it because she'd got another son and a daughter that could've done it if they'd have put their mind to it, but I did it because it would have fallen on my Mum if I hadn't have done it. So *yes I would* do that to help my parents out. I mean I'd do it for my grandmother but I'd do it to help them out. [Emphasis in original]

Janet seems unequivocal that she is doing this for her mother, because her mother is now in a position where she is *unable* to do as much for Doreen as before, but that the *proper* thing would be for her aunt or uncle to substitute in this way. It does not appear that Janet feels more obligated to her grandmother in particular than do her sisters – although that could perhaps change over time. What is being activated is her commitment to her mother, and her availability to help. She lives near to her parents, unlike her two sisters who live in other parts of the country.

The fourth way in which the overall pattern of commitments has been consolidated is a procedural matter, about how negotiations are conducted, and focuses upon Doreen's own position in the family. As time has passed, and the situation has developed, it has become more difficult for Stan and Eileen to raise the issue of responsibility for Doreen in open discussions. Although all our Simpson interviewees had obviously talked together about the unequal contributions made to supporting Doreen, no one had raised it with the siblings. Julie has her own explanations for this:

> *Julie* I don't think really Mum and Dad have pushed it as much as they could do. If they really wanted to push it I think they could and, it would be done very grudgingly [laugh] I think, but at least it would be done. It's rotten because, for my grandmother, I mean you have to keep it from her that you're having trouble getting people to look after her obviously. But

I think she knows really that they don't really pull their weight, its just she gets very protective if you start saying that they should do this, this and this. I don't really know what they can do about it. To say to somebody 'You've got to have her this weekend' then she feels like she's a parcel you're passing around which isn't very fair. That's part of the reason why Mum and Dad haven't really pushed it very much because they feel its rotten for her to feel she's a burden to anybody.

What Julie is saying – and this is reflected also in other people's comments – is that they have found it impossible to address openly the question of the difficulties now arising, because Doreen's feelings would be hurt.

Again her comments point to the likelihood that open discussion would make Doreen feel too dependent ('she feels she's like a parcel you're passing around'). As we indicated in Chapter 2, maintaining the balance between dependence and independence can be as much a matter of how these issues are *treated* in negotiations, as the actual balance of losses and gains in material terms. Open discussion of itself would make no difference to the pattern of giving and receiving help. The problem with it is that it would make it impossible for Doreen to sustain a view of herself as having giving and receiving held roughly in balance. Open discussion would also call into question the moral reputation of her other children – a matter of considerable importance in family relationships, we shall argue in Chapter 5. In examples like this it becomes clear why people sometimes do not engage in open discussion, despite the fact that they value it as a way of sorting things out. But the fact that they could not discuss the matter openly also had the effect of limiting the room for manoeuvre which Stan and Eileen had, and therefore shaped the way in which their actions developed.

These then are the four strands which we can detect in the story of how commitments had developed in the Simpson family over the past eighteen years. They enable us to explain the pattern of family responsibilities accepted by different parties at the time of our interviews. They enable us to make sense, for example, of why it was becoming an important yet apparently an unresolvable problem for Stan and Eileen to negotiate a different division of responsibilities.

Negotiations about family responsibilities in the Simpson case

What does the Simpson case tell us about our two key themes in this chapter: negotiations and developing commitments?

First, in the Simpson family, the responsibilities accepted were clearly a product of negotiation rather than of following rules of obligation. Stan's and Eileen's commitment to Doreen cannot be explained by the rule-following model. If Stan's action in offering Doreen a home was a simple expression of rules of filial obligation, then why did not the same rules apply to his siblings? And if the development of Eileen's own commitment to Doreen expressed gendered rules of obligation which specify that women should look after relatives, then why did that not apply first to Doreen's daughter?

Of course rules are not always followed – they can be acknowledged in principle but broken in practice. But we do not think that this explanation really fits our case. Certainly none of our interviewees talked in this way. Rather we are arguing that the commitments, as well as the precise ways in which these were fulfilled at different times, had been negotiated over time. Implicit negotiations about commitments were taking place gradually, between individuals, sometimes over many years, *as well as* more explicit negotiations from time to time about how these should be fulfilled. Thus by the time Doreen needed support following the death of her husband, it had already become obvious to Stan that he, rather than his siblings, would take the responsibility. But his commitment to Doreen had developed through a relationship with her which had been negotiated implicitly between them over many years, and over many exchanges of support. Eileen's commitment to Doreen began to develop once the conditions were right; so too did Janet's involvement with her grandmother, because of her commitment to her parents. All these strands in the Simpsons' story show how responsibilities build up incrementally over time through quite complex processes in exchange relationships. This seems less a 'given' of specific genealogical relationships, than a product of negotiations within certain social conditions.

Also we can see here that the products of negotiations – and in essence what was being negotiated about – were not simply the exchanges of material assistance, but also moral aspects of identities and responsibilities. The siblings, Stan, Eileen and Doreen, all were gaining moral reputations in each others' eyes as well as moral responsibilities *through* the way they negotiated and dealt with their relationships with each other. These in turn informed the way negotiations continued. For example, Stan and Eileen were influenced by their view of the siblings' conduct in considering how best to involve them in supporting Doreen. They were also constrained by it from discussing the question openly. In that sense, even apparently moral dimensions of the situation could have material as well as moral outcomes, because they influenced the continuing pattern of material support.

Our second main point is about implicit and explicit negotiations. In the Simpson case, where we have a great deal of detail, we can see that both were used. Explicit negotiation is always easier to describe and certainly they used it. Indeed the idea and practice of explicit negotiation comes through as something valued highly by our Simpson interviewees – it is particularly clear in Stan and Eileen's relationship to their daughters, which we have not discussed here. However, it is also clear that explicit discussions about kin support were set within more implicit processes which took place over time. So, although the Simpsons certainly did negotiate explicitly about various types of support, that was only ever part of the negotiating process.

There are a number of ways in which this can be demonstrated. As with some other examples earlier in this chapter, open discussions did not invariably include everyone relevant. To understand the role of such people we need to be aware of more implicit negotiations. The most obvious examples of people excluded in this way are the siblings and Doreen herself. This might mean a number of things. For example, the positions and responsibilities of people who do not participate may already have been implicitly negotiated, so that 'everybody knows' about it, without having to have a discussion. Certainly, on this basis Stan and Eileen have not yet attempted to include his siblings in negotiations about helping Doreen. A similar explanation, focusing on non-decision-making, could account for a complete absence of discussion about what to do, or who should do what. Alternatively, the exclusion of certain people may have arisen because their inclusion would influence the moral outcomes of the negotiation. Stan and Eileen, for example, felt that the offer of a home for Doreen should come from them, so that she did not have to ask for help and compromise her independence. On that basis, they excluded her from discussions until the offer was made. Similarly, we have suggested, she was excluded from subsequent discussion because again it would have been too difficult to include her without overturning her position in the dependence–independence balance.

There are other possibilities, but the general point about all of these explanations is that explicit discussions at any one time are likely to be only the tip of the iceberg of negotiations which have taken and are taking place, and really only make analytical sense if we can see the implicit negotiations simultaneously. Certainly, if we want to know about how certain patterns of kinship responsibility come about, then focusing on explicit discussions is not enough. This is not to deny the importance of explicit negotiations, however. Indeed they carry their own distinctive implications. We note, for example, that Stan's siblings felt able to hold Stan and Eileen responsible for the outcome of their decision to offer Doreen a home, and felt themselves absolved of overall responsibility for her, precisely because they had been openly consulted and had made their views public.

Our third main point from the Simpson case is that it confirms the importance of building the perspective of time into our analysis. The processes through which negotiations occur, as well as their outcomes, have lasting implications. Through negotiations people create sets of material and moral baggage which get carried forward, and which help to create the framework for future negotiations. Material baggage is perhaps most easily recognised, as the actual exchanges of goods and services which occur over time, and which help to constitute people's material positions *vis-à-vis* other kin. Moral baggage, on the other hand, is less tangible, but involves the moral identities and reputations of the participants also constructed through this process. Explicit negotiations in the Simpson family did implicate people's moral identities, for example Stan's siblings being 'not above refusing'. In this sense moral identities were produced and reshaped through negotiations, as well as giving shape to the form the negotiations took.

We think that it is the accumulation of moral and material baggage which is the key to understanding what negotiation means in practice – whether or not it is explicit – and how commitments between kin are forged. If we wish to understand the bargaining stances people can take in negotiations about commitments to their kin we believe that it is vital to take account of these moral dimensions of negotiations and of commitments built up over time. It is not sufficient to focus simply on the material value of exchanges which have taken place. We develop this view in slightly different ways in Chapter 5.

THE CONCEPT OF COMMITMENT IN FAMILY RESPONSIBILITIES

At this point in our discussion we want to focus our analysis on the concept of commitment, which we have used extensively in this chapter. We believe that it is a fruitful way of conceptualising family responsibilities. The process of negotiating these responsibilities, we have argued, is one through which commitments develop and emerge. Over time, one individual becomes committed to giving certain forms of help to another, or to responding positively to any such requests which may be made in the future. In this sense commitments are the products of negotiations.

We find the concept of commitment a useful way of thinking about this for various reasons. It enables us to emphasise that the exchanges of goods and services are not reckoned purely in material terms, but also have moral dimensions. It also enables us to emphasise the seriousness of the way in which people approach these aspects of family relationships, and the significance of the personal consequences which can flow from them. We have argued against the idea that these are 'rules of obligation' which people follow. But an absence of rules does not mean that these aspects of family life are marginal or unimportant, or that people may lend a hand to relatives from time to time but this has little effect on the rest of their lives. Our use of the term commitment is meant to convey that much more is going on than simply 'doing the tasks'. But the idea of 'rules' is the wrong way to look at it.

Commitments represent responsibilities accepted which have real and lasting consequences. And commitments developed oneself through one's own negotiations with others are likely to feel much more powerful than rules imposed from 'outside'. The fact that someone is actively shaping the course of their own relationships, rather than following externally imposed rules, thus binds them in the more tightly. It is important therefore to understand that people do see themselves as having choices about which direction to go in, even if those choices are constrained at any point in time by other choices which they have made in the past. When we talk about commitments 'accumulating' over time we do not mean to imply that more and more responsibilities build up in a process over which the individual has no control. As we noted earlier in this chapter, respondents to our survey did not approve of the characters in our vignette just taking on more and more responsibility for elderly parents without considering other factors in their lives. Our interview data bear out that, in practice, people do see themselves as actively constructing their own commitments, in a process over which they have some measure of control – albeit rather limited in certain cases.

These points can be seen clearly in our case study of the Simpson family. We are able to see Stan and Eileen's actions over a period of nearly twenty years. We see them taking a series of steps, each of which draws them in more closely to a particular form of commitment to Stan's mother. Each step closed off certain options for the future and opened up others. The steps which they took also affected the form of commitment which Stan's siblings developed for their mother. In turn, the path along which the siblings moved affected what Stan and Eileen could do. By the time we interviewed them, Stan and Eileen felt that their room for manoeuvre was very limited, so firmly had they become set on a particular path. However, another set of renegotiations *was* beginning to take place. We doubt that we can ever say that a point has been reached where a set of commitments becomes totally fixed, immovable, non-negotiable. But some people's situation comes fairly close to that, and can certainly *feel* like that – as did Stan and Eileen's.

In thinking about analysing our own data on these issues, and in thinking about their wider significance, we have found Howard Becker's work on the concept of commitment very helpful (Becker, 1960). Although he does not specifically discuss responsibilities of kinship, he does develop the idea that commitments between people get consolidated over time. A key element in understanding this process, he argues, is that commitments get consolidated because it becomes too expensive for people to withdraw from them. Becker argues that people make investments or 'side bets' which they would lose if they failed to continue on a committed path. These side bets are often made implicitly through 'a series of acts no one of which is crucial but which, taken together, constitute for the actor a series of side bets of such magnitude that he [sic] finds himself unwilling to lose them' (Becker, 1960: 38). Thus commitments may develop gradually over time, but equally may also get consolidated or shaped through explicit renegotiations. The importance of this is that it emphasises the potential of past actions and negotiations to become the context for future choices, or indeed the very fabric of constraint and opportunity from which choices are fashioned through negotiations. Negotiation, in that sense, is never 'structure-less' or free, but equally it is not determined by structure or by fixed rules of conduct.

For us, one of the strengths of Becker's analysis is his concept of 'valuables' created through this process of side-betting. These valuables can be measured in both material and moral terms. Therefore, just as someone may lose out materially by withdrawing from a relationship based on the exchange of material resources, so too they may lose a valuable reputation if they withdraw support and let someone down. And these moral valuables need to be understood in their cultural context, so that what is considered to constitute a good reputation for a woman in our society may differ from the constituent parts of a good reputation for a man. Becker uses the example of chastity to illustrate this. In relation to family responsibilities, we are concerned with different types of reputation (as we indicate in Chapter 5) but his argument certainly can be applied. The important point is that, in order to understand whether or not someone is 'committed', we need to be sensitive to the full range of losses that person feels they would make by withdrawing from a path on which they have begun. These are the valuables which have the effect of locking someone into a particular set of responsibilities, progressively over time.

CONCLUSION

In summary, the material in this chapter confirms both the importance of negotiations as the way in which family responsibilities are developed, and also the complexities of the processes involved in this. Not only do people actually negotiate their family responsibilities in practice, but they also see this as the *proper* way to proceed. Both in responding to survey questions, and in their own relationships, negotiating is seen as entirely appropriate.

The fact that the responsibilities which people accept are negotiated – rather than the consequence of following rules of obligation – clarifies why there is such variation in practice. People in apparently similar positions (even within the same family) come to accept very different levels and types of responsibility precisely because these are negotiated individually. However, the responsibilities which do develop in this way are real and significant in people's lives – and for those who develop extensive responsibilities they can be extremely significant. We have argued that the concept of 'developing commitments' is a helpful way of understanding this. One's gender, and one's genealogical relationship to others, may be relevant in the way that commitments develop. However, we do not think that the idea that people follow rules based on categories of gender or genealogy is particularly plausible as an explanation. Instead, we have suggested that the social conditions under which gender and genealogy are lived may help to create conditions which are conducive to the development of certain kinds of commitments between individuals. Ultimately, though, those commitments are *created* not *ascribed*.

We have been able to show that the actual process of negotiation takes many forms. Implicit negotiation forms the backcloth, and in a sense is proceeding all the time as people meet, talk and relate to each other. Sometimes it is supplemented by explicit negotiations, sometimes not. The process of weaving together different forms of negotiation is complex and elaborate, but seems to be well understood by the participants. We have suggested that this indicates that there may be guidelines about procedures (that is, about how to negotiate, and what factors can be taken into account) even if there are not discernible rules about the substance of responsibilities. Certainly, people do make judgements about each others' behaviour in negotiations, and form ideas about what is legitimate and what is not. This issue is considered more fully in the next chapter.

4   Making legitimate excuses

INTRODUCTION: UNDERSTANDING LEGITIMATE EXCUSES

In the last chapter we explored the concept of negotiation and looked at the complex processes through which patterns of commitment had developed over time in one kin group. We suggested that negotiations are never sequences of completely separate events: both moral and material elements are carried forward into subsequent negotiations. We argued that *the way* people negotiate can have just as enduring a significance as the material outcomes of negotiations. This occurs because, through the process of negotiation, people construct social meanings which help everyone to make sense of the past, present and future. In this chapter we develop further our analysis of the way social meanings are constructed and deployed. We do this by focusing on a particular set of 'meanings', which we are calling 'legitimate excuses'.

Our focus on 'legitimate excuses' enables us to understand dimensions of the process of negotiating family responsibilities which were somewhat muted in Chapter 3. We were concentrating then on the processes through which people become committed to another person, and to providing assistance when they need it. But we have also noted throughout this book that there is great variation in the extent to which people provide help for their kin, or feel that they 'ought to' do so. So it is just as important to understand the processes involved in *not* becoming committed. The concept of 'legitimate excuses' represents our main organising theme for exploring this. In its crudest form, what we want to know is whether and how some people can legitimately avoid becoming committed. Is non-commitment sanctioned in some circumstances but not in others? Or for some people but not for others? Do people ever consciously and actively avoid becoming obligated? Although the term 'excuses' implies a kind of illicit avoidance of obligation, we are using it in a wider and non-judgemental sense to look at justificatory accounts which get deployed within negotiations, and how legitimacy gets constructed within that context.

In exploring this issue, we turn first to our survey data. At the level of public norms, there is evidence that people recognise different types of justificatory account. In general it seems that people accept more readily that it is legitimate for someone to refuse help to a relative if they are unable to provide assistance, rather than able but unwilling. This contrast between 'unable' and 'unwilling' runs through answers to our survey questions and is also reflected in our interview data. For example, in the survey, in response to the question 'Are there any circumstances in which it is reasonable to refuse to provide personal help for a sick or elderly relative?', 58 per cent of our respondents answered yes, and 37 per cent said no. This is not a clear consensus (our consensus baseline was 75 per cent). However, the 58 per cent who had answered 'yes' to the first part of the question were asked under what circumstances it would be reasonable to refuse (an open-ended, post-coded question), and they gave answers concentrated around the following themes: having other prior commitments, not being available, not being able because of lack of skill, physical incapacity or geographical distance (76 per cent of responses fell into these categories taken as a whole). We had no evidence that different categories of respondent were answering in different ways, except a slight tendency for women to emphasise commitments to 'one's own family', and men to emphasise 'employment'.

The concept of ability (or inability) to give help seems to be important at the level of public norms, in constructing justificatory accounts of one's own actions or other people's. But how does ability or inability get defined? If it is so important to establish that you are unable rather than unwilling to help, is it important to get that definition of the situation accepted by other people? What are the limits to this? These are key questions which we try to answer in this chapter.

An example from one of our kin groups helps to raise some of the important issues which we are considering in this chapter. It concerns the Mansfield family, and we are using material from our interview with Roger Mansfield where he discusses some of the negotiations which took place around the care of his father, who died some years previous to our interviews (we have also discussed aspects of this case study in Finch and Mason, 1990b). Although we interviewed other members of the Mansfield family, we are simply using extracts from Roger's interview to introduce some of the important themes concerning legitimate excuses. Roger told us that, initially, he and two of his sisters took most of the responsibility for his father's care. At the time, Roger was a mature student studying for a degree, and was married with young children. He explained the circumstances like this:

Roger I was at University at the time so it was [laugh] it wasn't too bad, I could get the time.

Interviewer You were flexible?

Roger Yes, and my two sisters didn't work so obviously they had, although they had young families they could fit it in whereas, the eldest two sisters, one was working full-time, the other one owned a business, so it was much more difficult for them.

Although Roger was apparently 'flexible', it emerged later in his interview that accommodating the care of his father was actually rather difficult, because he had quite a heavy workload as a student, and was in the process of taking university examinations. Roger explained that there was a 'certain resentment' because not everybody got equally involved. Some members of the family claimed they were *unable* to provide practical support because of employment and business commitments. However, they were not fully successful in getting this accepted by the rest of the family. Since they felt unable to provide time and labour, they offered financial support, but from Roger's point of view, this was not an acceptable alternative.

Roger Course they threw money at the problem you see, that was another way. Because they own businesses sort of 'Money's no object, take that' [laugh] its, a sort of way of saying 'Well I can't help but you know I'll supply money for whatever's needed.' They could have had anything they wanted [laugh].

Interviewer But that's not quite the same you think?

Roger No. Well it was useless to anybody. He had money of his own anyway. That wasn't what he needed. It was care and attention I suppose.

Nevertheless, both the resentment, and the feeling that the excuses were illegitimate, were not made public to the whole family or voiced explicitly to the 'miscreants'. But there was a sense in which everybody knew.

Roger I don't think anyone ever is really very confident to say 'Hey, you know, I think I'm getting the raw end of this deal.' They tend to sort of form little groups to [laugh] complain among themselves. I don't think it ever came out in the open, but there again I think everybody *knew* you know [laugh].

However, as Roger's father Vic's condition became worse, and he was hospitalised, a further complication emerged. Vic was unhappy in hospital, and wanted to come home. This prompted a set of negotiations in which the legitimacy of excuses did get openly discussed.

Roger He [father] wanted to stay in his own house but [pause] that would mean somebody living with him. But we all had our own houses and things. We were all married and all had our own houses, families and all the rest of it [pause and sigh]. The only solution really was that my mother went back.

Roger's mother, Nan, was the only one without a legitimate excuse at that time. When it actually came to taking Vic into one of their homes, the sibling group appeared to accept that none of them were able to do this. Nan did offer an excuse: she had been estranged from Vic for several years. So why did her excuse look less credible? This is what Roger says:

> *Roger* I explained the situation to her, I said 'Well I think the only solution is that you go back home' so she hit the roof, went mad, told me I didn't know what I was talking about and all the rest of it and I said 'Well having said all that, I still feel that its your responsibility.' I said '*We* can't do it, you know, for various reasons.' I told her all the reasons I felt we *couldn't* do it and she said 'No I won't do it' so I said 'Well as far as I'm concerned you should do it', I said, 'and furthermore I think we're all of the opinion that you should.' You see I know my mother and the only way was to put pressure on her as, as a sort of group [laugh]. [Emphasis in original]

Taken as a whole, we think that what Roger Mansfield tells us raises a number of important themes concerning legitimate excuses. First, it does confirm that legitimacy hinged upon being able to claim inability rather than unwillingness to provide support. Certain factors, for example being at home with young children, or having the 'flexibility' of a student, apparently made Roger and his sisters look available and able to help.

Second, however, the situation was not totally clear-cut. The ability or inability of each relative to offer help had to be *established*. In the process excuses clearly got deployed and accepted with varying degrees of success. For example, the siblings with full-time employment and their own businesses looked less available to help by comparison with the others, but perhaps not so unavailable as to be able to provide no help at all. In that sense, excuses really are meanings which are getting constructed and deployed within negotiating processes. Certainly, when Nan was drawn into the negotiations, Roger actively drew a distinction between the legitimacy of the excuses of himself and his siblings in comparison with hers. He based this very much on their *inability* to help, as compared with her *unwillingness*. His account places emphasis on the words 'we can't' 'you should', and on the fact that he is able to claim that the sibling group were all agreed on the illegitimacy of Nan's position.

Third, as we might expect given our arguments about negotiations in the previous chapter, excuses can be constructed and deployed implicitly as well as explicitly, and their legitimacy can be contested or affirmed at both levels too. Just as with the development of commitments, in many instances excuses and their legitimacy may be unspoken, having developed over time, and may be taken for granted by, or known to, all participants.

Fourth, the ability to get an excuse accepted as legitimate clearly did not depend straightforwardly on what the excuse was, or on who was offering it, although both of these factors were relevant. What comes across as more important in the Mansfield case is the set of circumstances under which excuses were getting mobilised by the various participants. For example, initially – when the issue under negotiation was the short-term care of Vic – some of Roger's siblings' excuses were not entirely accepted as legitimate. But later on, once the circumstances changed and the issue became one of what to do on a more permanent basis, it was Nan's excuse which came into focus, and lost its earlier legitimacy. At that stage, the sibling group mobilised the idea that Nan had a stronger responsibility than they did to care for her ex-husband.

However, there are two reasons why we think it would be wrong to suggest that the Mansfield case is an example of the operation of a genealogical or gender hierarchy according to which excuses will be accepted or rejected (see Finch and Mason, 1990b). First, if it was always the case that a wife's excuse was less likely than a son or daughter's to be accepted as legitimate, then why was Nan not put on the spot at an earlier stage? Similarly, if sisters' excuses are always less legitimate than those of their brothers, then why did Roger's full-time student status not legitimately excuse him from helping in the early stages? The idea of a genealogical or gender hierarchy does not directly account for what happened in the Mansfield example. Our second point is less concerned with whether empirical outcomes actually match up to the supposed hierarchical ordering of obligations, and more with the way in which the hierarchy is thought to influence the negotiating process. We *do* think the idea of a genealogical hierarchy had some relevance in the Mansfield negotiations. However, we see the process as one whereby meanings – which at certain times included meanings about a hierarchical ordering of obligations – were constituted and deployed in negotiations. Looked at in this way, it is not so much that a hierarchy was followed, but more that the *idea* of a hierarchy was *constituted* and *deployed* by some members of the family (that is, Roger and his siblings) as a lever in negotiations which were about the legitimacy of excuses.

Finally, the examples hint at a rather complex relationship between deploying an excuse that is legitimate, and deploying an excuse that *works* or has efficacy. For example, Roger's siblings deployed excuses about employment and other commitments which, by Roger's account, were not accepted as wholly legitimate. However, the excuses did work in the sense that they enabled those people to absent themselves from providing practical support without having too much overt pressure put on them. In strictly material terms then, the excuses worked, and the siblings escaped involvement in these particular transactions of practical support, even though their excuses were not accepted fully. This raises the question of whether legitimacy *matters*: as long as you have an excuse, does it really matter whether or not you can get it widely accepted that it is a legitimate one? We think that legitimacy does matter, and that people strive for it in their negotiations, because of its association with moral worth and identity.

EXCUSES AND THEIR USES

These then are the kinds of themes we are going to explore in this chapter. We are going to reject the position that the legitimacy of an excuse is a straightforward outcome either of *what* the excuse is, or of *who* is making the excuse. Although both of these factors are relevant, they do not determine outcomes straightforwardly. We are going to begin with a discussion of the range and types of excuses we discovered, drawing on both our qualitative and survey data sets. Following that, we will go on to examine the processes through which excuses get constituted as legitimate or otherwise, and the implications of this.

We have suggested that you will improve your chances of an excuse being regarded as legitimate if you can get it accepted as widely as possible that you are *unable* to help, rather than unwilling. The Mansfield case is an illustration of that. But, more generally, how can someone establish successfully that they are 'unable' to help? What grounds are likely to be accepted as good reasons for this inability?

Our interview data suggest that there is quite a wide variety of grounds on which someone can establish that they are unable to help. In this section we are going to give an overview of this variation. In effect, we are documenting the principles which people used in the processes of negotiating commitments and responsibilities in their own families. But we are leaving specific discussion of these processes until the following section. We can link the principles to our survey material too, to see how far these are factors which commend themselves to a statistically representative sample as constituting grounds for being unable to help a relative.

Employment

We begin with employment as a possible reason for being unable to help a relative. In our survey, we included three questions which asked directly about whether a person should give up a job to provide personal care for a relative. A consensus that people should not give up their jobs in these circumstances would suggest that, at the level of publicly expressed views, employment is seen as a legitimate excuse for inability to provide personal care. In fact, the pattern of responses we received does point in that direction, but is not straightforward or unequivocal.

In each of these examples, the question about giving up employment was part of a sequence of events and choices set out in our vignettes about Jim and Margaret Robertson (see Chapter 3), Jane and Ann Hill (see Chapter 2), and Valerie and Mary Harper (see also Chapter 2, and to be discussed more fully in Chapter 5). At some point in each vignette we made one or more characters face the choice of giving up paid work. Our survey respondents were asked to say if they should do so or not. The frequencies are set out in Table 4.1. None of the examples gives us a clear consensus (in terms of our consensus baseline) that it is absolutely legitimate to put a job before personal care of a relative, but the implication is that this *may* be legitimate. The impression is that the particular circumstances of each case govern how far employment would be widely accepted as a legitimate excuse. It is least widely accepted in the case of Jane Hill who (as we showed in Chapter 2) was locked into an ongoing relationship of practical material aid with Ann, and had substantial past assistance to reciprocate. However, reciprocating for past help – of a different kind – was not apparently such a significant factor in the pattern of responses in the Harper vignette. In that vignette, respondents had already been told that the grandmother had paid for a house deposit for her grand-daughter, when they were asked to decide whether the grand-daughter should give up her job. In this case people may have been swayed by the fact that it was a much younger woman who would be giving up a job – employment may be more readily accepted as a legitimate excuse for the young than for the middle-aged, especially women.

Our main point in comparing these examples is not to discuss the details of each vignette, but to illustrate that specific circumstances do seem to be crucial in determining whether employment is acceptable as a legitimate excuse. They also seem to override any consideration of genealogical 'closeness'. The person who, in the judgements of our survey respondents, will have most difficulty in getting this excuse accepted is Jane Hill, in respect of her *former* mother-in-law: a relationship which is tenuous, at best, in genealogical terms.

Turning now to our interview data, we can ask: to what extent in practice do people use employment as an 'excuse' for being unable to provide support? Does it only apply to personal care, or can the excuse of employment be used more widely? In fact, employment is the most common reason given for being unable to provide support in our qualitative data set. We have at least seventy accounts where employment, or less commonly

Table 4.1 Giving up employment to provide personal care

Jim and Margaret

Yes, Jim or Margaret should give up their job to care for Jim's widowed father:	22%
No, neither should give up their job:	64%

Jane and Ann Hill

Yes, Jane should offer to give up her job to look after her former mother in law, Ann:	43%
No, she should not give up her job:	41%

Valerie and Mary Harper

Yes, Mary's granddaughter should give up her job to look after Mary:	29%
No, the granddaughter should not give up her job:	57%

(Consensus baseline: 75%)

full-time study, were put forward as factors which influence the ability to provide assistance. Our examples cover several types of support, but the demands of one's job was most commonly cited as a reason for being unable to provide labour or time-intensive types of support. This included general practical help, child care and babysitting, and personal care. It was also commonly used to explain a failure to visit relatives very often, or to maintain general contact with them by telephone or letter. In all these cases people said that their job left them *insufficient time* to provide help, so it is not surprising that the support in question is clustered in the labour-intensive forms.

In considering the way in which employment 'works' as an excuse, it is important to recognise that it is not a factor whose effects are fixed or unambiguous. There is room for variation in whether someone sees a job, even a full-time job, as presenting an insurmountable barrier to spending time in helping a relative. We saw this to an extent in the example of the Mansfields. It also comes through clearly in the following example from Jean Crabtree, a woman in her twenties. In the following extract, Jean was telling us about the organisation of personal care for her maternal grandparents, which had taken place several years before:

Interviewer   Did you children get enlisted in any of that?
Jean   To some extent yes. I mean obviously we couldn't do as much because we were working and my sister had the family to look after, but we did visit them regularly and we did go and help, you know when we had the opportunity to, but it was my mum who did most of the work

helping them. And then her brother helped as well to some extent let's say. He was working, so obviously he couldn't do as much.

Interviewer And your mother was working part-time then was she, or . . . ?

Jean When my grandma and grandad were ill, she did give up work for some time to go and look after them, yeah. She didn't actually stay with them, but she went in the daytime and she also was the one responsible for, she went round social services organising home help and Meals on Wheels.

Jean's account shows a difference in the extent to which employment was viewed as prohibiting the provision of help. Although full-time employment prevented some of them from helping, her mother moulded the caring around her employment, and eventually gave up her job for a time. In that sense, she made herself available, or manipulated her own ability to provide support, rather than viewing inability as insurmountable.

We have many examples of people – unlike Jean's mother – viewing employment unproblematically as a factor preventing involvement in responsibilities to kin. Here is one where the young man involved (coincidentally he is Jean Crabtree's partner) has operated with this kind of reasoning, and has become rather isolated from the regular exchange of practical and financial support, and the family business, which characterise his large family of origin (see Appendix A – the Crabtree kin group – for details). It is interesting that he begins to reflect on the legitimacy of his position in the interview.

David Waterworth It would be very difficult, well it would be very difficult to actually get involved because I've got other commitments.

Interviewer I'm sure, of course I can see that. But it's quite interesting, because you're the eldest child, in fact you're the eldest son, and some people would say in a family business, the eldest son really is the one who should sort of be involved in and take responsibility for [pause] there's never been any of those ideas around? [laugh] No?

David No, none whatsoever, because the career that I'm in takes up all my time and more besides, and I'm very devoted to that. So, er, its very much, I don't know, in some ways I feel guilty that I don't put as much time and effort, and help them out as I should do, because I feel my responsibilities you see. I have morals [laugh]. But whether the opportunity's actually arisen for me to, or whether I should make those opportunities arise and say 'Look what can I do to help?', maybe I should do that.

Other family commitments

The next 'excuse' which we shall consider is 'other family commitments'.
The clearest part of our survey which posed a choice between one set of
family commitments and another was in the vignette about Jim and Margaret
Robertson. At one point respondents were asked whether Jim and Margaret
should move to live near Jim's parents even though this might have a bad
effect on their teenage children's education. We got a clear consensus that
Jim and Margaret should stay where they were: 78 per cent said stay, 20 per
cent said move (consensus baseline 75 per cent). This is not the same as
saying that Jim and Margaret should give Jim's parents no help at all, but it
is a fairly clear message that it is legitimate for them to put their children first
over the question of whether or not to move.

In our qualitative data set, there are at least twenty-seven examples where
people's other family commitments are brought in as a factor relevant to
working out whether they are available to assist a relative. Sometimes it is
deployed as a reason for not helping. But it can also work the other way
round. In Jean Crabtree's example cited above, the fact that her sister had
young children was used as a reason why she could not get heavily involved
in giving personal care to her grandparents. Yet in Roger Mansfield's
example, given at the beginning of the chapter, the fact that two of his sisters
were at home with young children made them look more, rather than less,
available to care for their father. This is the more common pattern, and it
does tend to differentiate men and women since it is usually women who are
in the position of being at home with young children.

In general, the most common circumstances under which commitments
to one's 'own family' emerge as an excuse in our data set are, as with
employment, when there is a need for personal care or practical support. It
can also be relevant to the responsibility to visit relatives or just to keep in
contact. However, the following extract demonstrates that the idea of
commitments to 'one's own family' can also be used as a convincing
demonstration of inability to provide financial help to other relatives.

Sara Anwar   Nobody helps financially in my family, I know that. Nobody
can afford to help another person financially because everybody's got
their own family, they've got their own children, their wife or whatever.
Interviewer   But would they help, for example, mothers to daughters, or
fathers to sons, or . . .
Sara   Um [pause] a son might if he can afford it, help his mother
financially. It depends how much he earns. It's on the earning actually, I
think if I earned about £200 or £300 per week, surely I can afford to
support my parents financially. But I don't, I only earn £50 a week so
[laugh] . . .

In cases like this, people are activating the idea that they have finite resources – be it time, money or labour – and that it is appropriate to use the principle of putting one's 'own family' first to prioritise claims made on them.

Competence

Other ways in which people explain their inability to provide help to relatives revolve around the issue of competence. We did not have one specific survey question which addressed the issue of competence directly and exclusively, but in many of the questions it was one of a number of considerations. As we argued in Chapter 1, when the survey questions are taken together, a strong message which emerges is that people are more likely to accord responsibility to relatives when the assistance needed is *fairly limited* in terms of skill. Where a high level of skill is demanded – for example in questions implying that the person needs *nursing* care – more people said that state services were preferable to relatives. This implies that, at the level of public norms, people may consider a lack of competence or skill as a legitimate excuse for not helping relatives.

In our qualitative data set there were forty-two examples invoking a lack of a variety of competences as reasons why help could not be provided, or had to be limited. These included the lack of: expertise or experience, physical capacity, good health, 'natural' aptitude. These examples most commonly involved practical and personal help. We also had a few examples suggesting the existence of taboos about the giving and receiving of this kind of help.

As with employment, and with other family commitments, there is room for a great deal of variation in how far people see lack of competence as insurmountable and straightforwardly ruling out the provision of support. Similarly, there is variation in what degree of competence people feel is necessary for support to be provided adequately. Some people, like Lawrence Gardner in the following extract, push their ability to help rather a long way. Others more readily cite the possibility that helping may cause ill-health, or their lack of other competence as a reason for not taking on the responsibility in the first place.

> *Lawrence* I'm just speaking now because it's just happened to us lately you see because I've just lost my dad you see. That, that was you know, I stayed with him. I lived with him [while he was ill]. I lived with him you see until it was affecting *my* health you see, so then we had to get him away you see, that's why *we* turned to the state [pause]. We *did* do what we could until it was too much you see. I mean my sister is in ill-health herself you see, she's got angina, she couldn't you see, so, and she lives

away. So it was falling on me and Caroline [wife] you see, so er, they brought him here, and we took him home, and I stayed with him, and lived with him you see. It were only just over a month or so, but we couldn't do no more you see.

There is a gender dimension involved in the issue of competence. We had some examples where both men and women suggested that women were particularly good at certain kinds of family responsibilities – most notably acting as a family 'lynchpin' or 'kinkeeper', or providing personal care or emotional support. The Arkright kin group provides one such example (see Appendix A for kin group details). Our interviewees from this family included three brothers, and two sisters – all young adults. Interestingly, all the brothers suggested that women tended to be better at 'being caring', or 'motherly' as one of them, Oskar, put it. In particular though, when asked to anticipate what would happen if their parents (who were at the time fit and healthy) needed personal care, the brothers all felt that one or all of their sisters would take the lead role. Here is Eric Arkright's version:

> *Eric*   It's usually women that do that sort of thing. Don't mean to be sexist of course [laugh]. But if it was up to me I'd help if I could. But I mean you'd probably find that men aren't very good at um, looking after people. Well *I* wouldn't be any good at it anyway . . .
> *Interviewer*   Can you see someone, a member of the family, who would probably take most responsibility [in that kind of situation]?
> *Eric*   Yes, yes. Probably Simone, I imagine. Simone or Selina. I know *I* couldn't do it. I wouldn't know where to start and, I mean I'd help as much as I possibly can, but I don't think I could look after them all day.

Certainly, Eric's comment that 'It is usually women who do that sort of thing' holds for our qualitative data set. Appendix C shows that we have twice as many examples of women providing personal care as men. Simone, one of Eric's sisters, also recognised this to be the common pattern and, like her brothers, she saw women as more caring than men. However, she clearly viewed these skills as acquired through experience and practice, rather than seeing their absence as insurmountable. Her interview gives a sense that she feels both irritation that men do not cultivate the skills needed for personal care, but also a sense of inevitability that that is the way it is.

Geographical distance

Geographical distance is one of the most obvious possible excuses at a common-sense level for not helping a relative. If you live a long distance away, you can hardly be seen as available to give practical or personal help can you?

In our view, it is nothing like as simple as that. People's perception of the significance of distance can and does vary. In the survey, we asked what our respondents thought would be the longest reasonable time for someone to travel one-way each day to care for a sick or elderly relative. The responses were as follows:

Less than 15 minutes	12%
16–30 minutes	55%
31–45 minutes	8%
46–60 minutes	18%
Over one hour	6%

There is clearly no consensus here, although a majority of people specified a fairly short period of time. The clearest message we get from this is that it is very rare for people to see it as appropriate to spend over one hour travelling to provide care. Does this correspond with messages we get from our qualitative data set?

The answer to that question is a qualified yes. Certainly, geographical distance is very commonly used to explain the inability to provide support, or to visit relatives. We have fifty-two examples of this. Sometimes the distances involved can be quite short, whether measured in miles or in the amount of time or effort it takes to travel them. However, we also have a few examples of people travelling very long distances, or following complicated journeys, in order to fulfil responsibilities to relatives. Indeed, we cited one of these examples – Maureen Vickers and her mother – in the introductory pages of this book. Here are some examples to illustrate the range. The first involves a fairly typical and unremarkable case. Sally Brown is explaining why she, rather than her sister who lives some 30 miles away, has consistently been more involved in providing personal care and practical support for their parents.

> *Sally* She is very tied up in her own, her sons [pause] of course her family is spread out over so many years as well. And she has a little business. And she is very tied physically to Crewe.

In a fairly matter of fact way, Sally is listing a number of potential excuses for her sister, including geographical distance. Anna Yates in the following extract is explaining her own behaviour, and feels slightly more uncomfortable about it than did Sally about her sister's. She is talking about her relationship with her grandmother. Anna is fond of her grandmother, and has recently moved near to her since leaving her parents' home.

> *Anna* I wouldn't like to say I wish I could see more of her because that's an excuse. Before I was far away and I've moved here and don't see any

more of her, you know, which is a shame. I know I should. She's dying to come here again you know, but it's just getting round to invite her, and with not having a car it makes everything that bit more awkward, but we do have my husband's mum's car *every* weekend, so it's not a really very good excuse [laugh]. But with not driving myself . . . . (Emphasis in original)

Anna is clearly searching for more excuses, because geographical distance can no longer be offered as a convincing explanation of her limited contact with her grandmother.

A final example comes from Simone Arkright. She is talking about the extent to which her sister, who lives in Canada, continues to provide support for their parents despite the number of miles between them. Her sister has a lot of telephone contact with her parents, but also, as Simone explains:

Interviewer   Your older sister, presumably there would be limits on what she could do as she's in Canada?
Simone   Yes, yes, yes. But when she does come over she does spend the whole two weeks cleaning. Does the house top to bottom.

Geographical distance is perhaps one of the best ways to demonstrate that excuses are not objective 'things'. Some people will view 10 or 20 miles as prohibitive, while others will travel more than 200 miles to provide or rotate the provision of personal care. These differences cannot be explained solely in terms of relative access to private transport, since we have examples of people making complicated bus or train journeys and covering a larger number of miles that others – who have access to a car – view as prohibitive. Geographical distance is also a good example of a 'variable' which is certainly not an 'independent variable'. It is not straightforwardly 'out there' and insurmountable in everyone's reckoning. People can and do manipulate the distance at which they live from their kin. Our argument here is parallel with employment. Just as there is room for variation in how far people see *time* as a prohibiting factor, so there is similar variation in judgements about *distance*.

Lack of resources

Finally, we want to consider lack of resources as a potential excuse. As we have shown, this does actually run behind most of the others so that, for example, people may well be thinking about lack of time, or money, or access to private transport and so on when raising other issues. Again, we did not have a survey question which addressed this exclusively. However, as we noted in Chapter 1, in general we do get a message from our survey that people see it as relevant to consider whether the assistance required represents a necessity, or a luxury, in deciding whether relatives should help. People generally see it as perfectly legitimate for relatives to refuse to give assistance for luxury items, especially where this may result in hardship for the person helping. This suggests there is public recognition that the relative distribution of resources in a family is a relevant consideration in deciding the legitimacy of a refusal to give help.

In our qualitative data set we identified fifty-five examples where people were putting forward a lack of resources specifically as an explanation of inability to provide support. However, as with the other excuses, we cannot identify an objective *level* of resources which people agree is needed in order to provide support, and below which people will agree that this is not possible. On the contrary, there is a wide range across which people's views about the connection between resources and ability are cast. The lack of financial resources is commonly cited as an excuse, often in a very matter of fact way. For example, Zaki Jones makes the following comparison between his two grandmothers:

> *Zaki* My grandmother gave me £500 for my twenty-first birthday, which paid for my fare to the States.
> *Interviewer* That's nice, which grandmother?
> *Zaki* My mother's mother. That paid for the fare. She seems to have lots of shares and things which she occasionally sells [laugh] . . .
> *Interviewer* Does she sort of spend money on you regularly? I mean that was obviously a special kind of thing.
> *Zaki* Oh yes, she does. She frequently gives me a bit of money.
> *Interviewer* So that's not like a loan? You wouldn't ask her for a loan? She's just a bit generous to you?
> *Zaki* Yes, yes. Although she did say that if I did get an offer for a course next year at University, and didn't have a grant, then she would be prepared to partly finance it [laugh].

And later in the interview:

> *Interviewer* How about your other grandmother, does she . . .
> *Zaki* Well she can't afford to really. I mean she doesn't really have too much money to throw around.

Appendix C shows that Zaki's potential experience of receiving financial support from a grandmother for education would be a rare one in our data set. Out of fifteen examples of financial help for education, eleven were concentrated in the parent–child range. However, for Zaki, it was normal and reasonable that his wealthy grandmother should help in this way, and in general that one of his grandmothers was more able to provide financial help than the other.

In general, of course we cannot know where people draw a line between being able to afford to provide support, and not doing so, but we do have examples where we are certain that providing support involved financial or other hardship, yet people did not use this as a way of avoiding helping. Also, we have examples where people manipulated the resources they had to make it more possible to provide support, in situations where it may have been perfectly reasonable to claim inability. This could take the form, for example, of building a house extension to accommodate the support of a relative.

Taken together, employment, other family commitments, competence, geography and resources were the main excuses recounted to us by our interviewees for some people's inability to provide assistance in certain circumstances. There is much variation in types of excuse and in their use, both within and between the categories we have identified, and we have used examples to give a sense of the range covered. Now we are going to turn the focus on to the processes through which people try to get their excuses accepted as legitimate.

MAKING EXCUSES AND CONSTRUCTING MEANINGS

The previous section described a series of broad principles which people in our study used to determine whether it was possible to give help to a relative, and how their time, money and labour should be prioritised. However, we showed that what those principles mean when translated into practice is remarkably variable. In the remainder of this chapter we are going to focus directly on the processes through which 'excuses' get constructed and deployed, and how they come to be recognised as legitimate or illegitimate. We want to move our readers away from seeing excuses as straightforward principles for application, or *things*. The position we are rejecting is that rules of obligation determine whether an excuse is accepted as legitimate or not: for example, a son can use the reason 'I live too far away' as a legitimate excuse for not visiting his parents regularly, in a way that a sister could not, because different rules of obligation apply to daughters and sons. We are saying that this is *not* how legitimate excuses work. It is not as simple as that, as our data show. Instead, we are suggesting that excuses and their legitimacy only make sense if we see them as products of the negotiating processes in which they are located. Negotiations provide the 'mechanisms' through which they are constructed, and the 'locations' in which they operate.

Our perspective throws the focus away from the content of an excuse, and on to the question of 'getting your excuse accepted' which we raised earlier in the chapter. Specifically, we can address a number of questions about getting excuses accepted. Through what processes do people get their excuses accepted as legitimate (or fail to do so)? Does the ability to get excuses accepted as legitimate vary according to genealogical position, or according to gender? For example, do women have more difficulty than men in getting certain actions accepted as legtimate? Does legitimacy itself actually *matter*? We are going to consider each of these questions in turn.

Through what processes do people get their excuses accepted as legitimate?

In order to tease out processes through which people try to get excuses accepted as legitimate, we shall discuss data on four cases in turn, then draw out some general points. Our discussion also draws on the analysis presented in Chapter 3, about the processes through which commitments develop.

Example 1: the Mansfields

For our first example we return to the Mansfield case, discussed at the beginning of this chapter. We looked earlier at Roger Mansfield's account of the care of his elderly father, Vic, and saw there that the use of employment as a legitimate excuse was a point of conflict in this family. We got a slightly different version of events from another member of the sibling group – Lesley Trafford – one of the three who had their own businesses and who used employment as an 'excuse'.

> *Interviewer* When your father was ill before he died, the family, different members of the family helped to look after him in various ways. Did you get involved in that?
> *Lesley* No, not at all. Not that I didn't want to. I think I would have liked to have done but [pause] there seemed to be so many of us trying to do so much. It seemed silly. And they always know that I'm here all the time, I'm never away from this place [her business premises]. I never have chance to get away from it. But, but I think if I'd been at home all day, or had a part-time job or something, then definitely I would have got, I would very much have liked to get involved.

In her account, not only is Lesley stressing that she was unable, not unwilling, to help, but also that 'they always know' that she is constantly at her business. For her, 'they' provide the audience which ratifies or confers the legitimacy of her excuse, so 'they' are important people to convince. It is through the audience that the excuse can become legitimate. Convincing them depends upon a mixture of getting herself accepted as someone who does not avoid obligations ('I would very much have liked to get involved'), and getting into a position where she does not actually assist. This mixture is one which evolves as a consequence of negotiations which take place over time, and this particular set of negotiations was part of that process.

> *Roger* Some members of the family thought that, you know, the businesses should take second place during that time, er, obviously they thought that it couldn't and you get conflicts built up in that way, but it, it was as though it was pushed on some more than others [pause] you know. But there again, I would imagine that's true of any family, there are people more able at a given time to help than others.

Although Roger is saying that legitimacy was disputed in this case, he is also saying that he accepts – at least in part, or on one level, or at some times – that such excuses can be valid and a 'normal' part of family life. These uncertainties add weight to the idea that the very issue of legitimacy was – and still is – being negotiated by members of this family. So when we observe that legitimacy is disputed, this potentially means two things. It can mean that legitimacy of a person's position is a matter of dispute between *different individuals*. It can also denote that the actions of an individual may seem to have legitimate and illegitimate elements, in the eyes of their kin. She or he is offering a range of explanations, the legitimacy of which may be more or less plausible at different times, or in different contexts. Attempts to establish legitimacy take different forms at different times and to different audiences. What both versions of disputed legitimacy have in common is that they demonstrate that legitimacy itself is not a fixed and immutable quality of specific actions, explanations or even people.

Example 2: the Gardners

Tim Gardner's account of negotiations about the care of his dying grandfather gives another example of excuses whose legitimacy is disputed. His paternal grandfather had recently been ill, and hospitalised, and this had prompted a set of explicit discussions between Tim's parents, and his aunt and uncle, about where he should live once he was discharged from hospital. In fact, members of neither household wanted Tim's grandfather to move in with them, primarily because Tim's uncle on the one hand, and Tim's mother on the other (that is, his children-in-law) did not get on well with him. Eventually, it was agreed that Tim's parents would take him in, and convert their garage to provide the space to do so, even though Tim's aunt and uncle had plenty of room in their large house. In fact, the issue only ever remained a hypothetical one, because Tim's grandfather died in hospital – but not before certain excuses had been aired.

Tim   My auntie and uncle's house, it's turned out since [pause] they've gone on for years saying 'Oh no we're not going to have him.' They used to say this with my gran as well, um when she was like in her wheelchair and so on. The house they've got has got six bedrooms, they had two children who are both now married and moved away. So they're on their own in a six-bedroomed house, but it's, well as my auntie put it, it's not owned by them, it's the company owns it. Well my uncle's a Director of this company and the company bought it for him to live in years and years ago. They said, um, you know 'It's just you and your children, no one else.' So it's all hush-hush and so on from their point of view, so we don't know too much about it. But that seems the basic reason, plus the fact that my uncle *did not* want him in the house. [Emphasis in original]

Tim makes it rather clear that he regards his uncle as offering a flimsy excuse. If his parents, who also 'did not want him in the house', were able to make room for his grandfather, his aunt and uncle could have done something similar, especially since his uncle is a Director of the company which owns their house. Elsewhere his account gives a picture of his parents looking for ways to make it possible for them to provide accommodation and care. He presents them as people who do not avoid responsibilities, and this is rather in contrast with his aunt and uncle whom he views as having developed a history of avoiding responsibilities – first to his grandmother, then his grandfather. It is this reputation, accumulated over some years, which throws into question the legitimacy of their excuse, and jeopardises 'public' acceptance (that is, acceptance by Tim and his parents) of their claim to be primarily unable rather than unwilling to help. For Tim, their position is not improved by the slightly suspect veil of secrecy drawn over the 'hush-hush' arrangements involving the ownership and use of their house.

Example 3: the MacIntyres

Our next example concerns the relationship of one of the young adults in our study with his widowed father. Thomas MacIntyre was a single man in his mid-twenties. He lived alone in a rented flat in a different part of Manchester to his father, although very near one of his sisters. His story concerns the legitimacy of offering a different kind of support to the one which is really needed or wanted. This is a variation on a theme highlighted in the Mansfield case earlier, where Roger Mansfield was critical of his brother and sister for failing to provide care or practical support for their father and instead 'throwing money at the problem'. We get a similar message from Thomas – that doing something else will not count in the legitimacy stakes.

Interviewer   Has your father got involved with giving any of you [that is, Thomas and his siblings] any kind of support perhaps . . .
Thomas   Um, not really, no.
Interviewer   Financial or practical?
Thomas   Well he's, he's the sort of, he will financially [pause] you'll have to be my agony aunt for the next three or four minutes. He will financially [pause] um but when it comes to any resource, time or effort, he's um, I think he thinks that 'I've done all I can over the last 25–30 years, its up to them now' [pause] which I can understand but he [pause] if it's money involved, all it takes is to write a cheque or, you know, get the old visit to the bank and he's quite amenable to that. But if it means you know, setting aside some time, or putting some effort into something, he's not so keen.

Thomas is obviously disappointed in what he perceives to be his father's use of money as an excuse not to provide other – more valued by Thomas – forms of support. Yet in the next few minutes of his interview, Thomas went on to spell out some explanations on behalf of his father – we might even call this making excuses for him – as to why his time was limited:

Thomas   Getting away from the money, he's um, he's got a partner himself now [pause] and um he spends quite a lot of time with her when he's not working [pause] so [pause] his, like his time is a bit more limited. He's not that mobile, he doesn't have a car, um, so again that's another limitation.

There is a sense in which Thomas cannot quite decide, or has competing ideas, about whether or not to accept the legitimacy of his father's excuses, and this is similar to the meanings-under-construction message we got from the Mansfields. He understands his father's predicament, but he would probably be more satisifed if his father made a 'publicly' recognisable attempt – one which would be recognisable in negotiations that is – to overcome some of the obstacles. In a sense, Thomas wants his father to show himself as the kind of father who will expend time and effort if he can. Developing that kind of family reputation seems actually to be more important than whether or not material support does regularly pass between them.

Example 4: the Crabtrees

This example draws primarily on the account of one of our young adults, Jean Crabtree, of the involvement of her mother and uncle in the care of their elderly parents. We introduced this case earlier, as an example of the use of employment as an excuse. Jean's mother took overall responsibility for the care of her parents, while Jean's uncle did a lot less. At first, Jean explains the discrepancy as a consequence of employment: her uncle got less involved because he had a job. However, later we learn that Jean's mother also had a job, which she gave up for a brief period, so that she could care for her parents. Employment status alone did not explain the difference. Jean discussed in some detail the comparison between the assistance given by her mother and her uncle. We asked whether she thought her uncle was 'trying to get out of' the responsibility to his parents, or whether there was a different explanation.

> *Jean*   I think partly, because with his first wife he had an awful lot of trouble for years and years. They didn't get on at all and she was a bit um, mentally disturbed in a lot of ways, so he did have a lot on his plate in that respect, you know sort of trying to cope with his wife and such a large family, and the home. So he did have a lot of other things to consider as well as my grandma and grandad. And I don't, in a way, I don't really think *he* thought he was capable of helping for some reason. He, I mean, he used to go and visit them that type of thing, but he never seemed to take it much further. He didn't seem to feel that he was *able* to for some reason. He'd not really had a lot of close contact with them, for a long time, mainly while he was with his first wife. He used to visit them, I don't even think it was once a week, occasionally he'd visit them and take one or other of the grandchildren to see them, but so up until he left his wife, you know, he had little contact with them. [Emphasis in original]

This example shows very clearly that getting an excuse accepted as legitimate can depend upon a long sequence of events set in motion before the specific need arises, or the specific excuse is aired. For Jean's uncle and mother, the different patterns of each of their contact and support over many years with their parents helped to put Jean's mother in a position where she felt a commitment to assist them, and Jean's uncle in a position where he felt *unable* to help. It is not entirely clear if his position was accepted as legitimate by other members of the family. Probably it was up to a point, as Jean indicates when she refers to his various prior commitments. She certainly seems to feel more comfortable viewing him as a person who lacked confidence in his own ability to help, rather than one trying to evade his responsibilities.

We can see from this example that it is vital to take account of how people are locked into and out of sets of commitments which have developed over time if we are to grasp the ways in which apparently straightforward excuses – like the initial use of employment in this case – get deployed and gain legitimacy.

These four examples show that people gain or seek the stamp of legitimacy for their excuses through processes of negotiation with their relations (negotiation, that is, in its fullest sense, as described in Chapter 3). When we talk about people making excuses, we literally do mean *making* them, and it takes more than one person to make a *legitimate* excuse. An excuse is not inherently legitimate or illegitimate, and achieving legitimacy seems to rest on two main principles.

First, it is important to get it accepted through negotiations that you have prior claims on your time or resources. This means that there should be some 'public' form of acceptance, that is, the relevant audience must agree that they are convinced. However, this kind of 'going public' does not necessarily mean that excuses must be articulated and discussed, because implicit negotiation may do just as well as long as everybody knows about it. But it does mean that your reasons must be open to scrutiny in *some* way: that way may just as likely be that they have been obvious, and everyone has known and accepted them for some time, as that you spell them out verbally at any one time. Of course this may not always work: Lesley Trafford (of the Mansfield family) told us that her relatives all knew that she was constantly tied up with her work, but Roger Mansfield tells us that he and his siblings were not entirely convinced that this was good enough to excuse her from participating in her father's care. Tim Gardner's aunt and uncle had always maintained that they were unable to use their home to provide support for relatives other than their own children, yet again other relatives saw this as unconvincing. In that example, the fact that the deal was 'hush-hush' and not open to scrutiny by the relevant audience, made it less likely that the excuse would be accepted by them as legitimate. The important point to be taken from these examples is that it is the audience which holds the power to grant or withhold legitimacy.

Second, you need to get yourself accepted as someone who does not wilfully avoid responsibilities. If you have a 'good' reputation, then inability to provide support will more readily be sanctioned as legitimate and genuine. Again, this is a process which must take place over time, through sequences of negotiation about a variety of issues and the concomitant development of moral identities. It was clearly relevant in the Mansfield and Gardner examples; for example, Tim Gardner made a direct comparison between his parents – as people who do not avoid responsibilities – and his aunt and uncle, as people who do. Lesley Trafford emphasised that she would have loved to have helped out with her father's care, if she possibly could. Perhaps the most clear example of this, however, is in Thomas MacIntyre's comments about his father. Essentially, Thomas is saying that he *would* accept his father's excuses as legitimate if only he had proved himself as the kind of father who did not avoid putting time and effort into his responsibilities to his children. This is not the same as saying that Thomas wants his father to do more: he wants to be able to recognise him as the kind of father who would do more.

Obviously there is a relationship between the support people give or receive and the reputations they develop in the eyes of their relatives, but it is not one of direct equivalence (we discuss this further in Chapter 5). Nevertheless, for some of those who acquire good reputations through the development of *commitments* to members of their family (see Chapter 3), the expense of withdrawing from commitments may be a much more potent factor in the range of responsibilities they develop, than is their capacity to establish legitimate excuses should the need arise. In other words they get into a situation – as did Stan and Eileen Simpson in Chapter 3 – where their own ability to make a legitimate excuse no longer has much relevance to how they work out what to do in practice.

Both of the broad principles outlined above are concerned with meanings and reputations which may be – and often are – contested and disputed by kin members. Added to that, individual people themselves can hold apparently contradictory views about legitimacy. The issue that remains is not whether an excuse *really* is legitimate (that would wrongly imply that legitimacy is an objective property of particular kinds of excuse) but what meaning it is given in negotiations by the people who matter. But how far does gender, or genealogical relationship, influence this process? We will now address these questions.

Does the ability to get excuses accepted as legitimate vary by gender, or genealogical relationship?

The answer to both of these questions is a qualified yes. It is a 'yes' because there is a tendency in our data for women on the one hand, and people within the parent–child range on the other, to have excuses accepted less readily than men, or than more genealogically distant kin, respectively. As far as gender is concerned, this trend seems most prominent in relation to labour or time-intensive types of support. However, the 'yes' is qualified because these are tendencies, but not hard and fast rules. For example, we saw at the beginning of the chapter in the Mansfield kin group example that the idea of a gendered or genealogical hierarchy according to which excuses would be accepted would neither have predicted what happened in practice, nor pinpointed the kinds of processes that were occurring. Empirically in our data set we have many variations on such a view of hierarchy, and conceptually it does not help to explain the ways in which legitimate excuses are constructed and deployed. Instead of supposing that the likely acceptance of excuses can be read off straightforwardly from the genders or genealogical relationships of the members of a family, we think it is important to delve deeper, and to establish *what it is about gender or genealogy* that we are reading when we observe such patterns. This will help us to make sense both of the gendered or genealogical patterns, and also the apparent variations on these. The position we are rejecting therefore is that genealogy or gender determine whose excuses will be accepted as legitimate in any straightforward sense.

So what is the relevance of gender, or of genealogy, in the making of legitimate excuses? We are going to focus more on gender than genealogy here, partly because we have already discussed the latter in relation to the Mansfield example, but also because the analytical arguments in many ways are similar in both cases and we want to concentrate on drawing parallels between them.

We think it is important to understand the ways in which people get locked into developing commitments, and how these vary for men and women. As we argued in the previous section, some people manage to avoid developing commitments to their relatives, and therefore when a specific need arises they are more likely to be able to argue successfully that they are unable to help (although ironically the legitimacy of their position may depend on their maintaining a reputation as someone who does not flagrantly evade responsibilities). But *precisely who* gets locked into sets of commitments over time does have a gendered (as well as a genealogical) component, as we argued in Chapter 3. We think it is at this level that we should look for gender differences in the process of getting excuses accepted as legitimate. For example, if women are more likely than men to develop commitments to relatives, it follows that they may find it more difficult than men to establish that they are 'unable' to help by virtue of their employment, their lack of skill, their other commitments, or whatever. What this means is that when it comes to a specific need, and the possible range of excuses, men and women may have access to a different repertoire. This may have the result that they actually make *different excuses* (because the same excuses would not make sense in relation to their relative biographies and contexts), or that they make the *same kinds of excuses but under different conditions*. But either way, when we are comparing men's and women's excuses in these situations, we are not comparing like with like.

The example of Jane Smith and her brothers helps to illustrate these points. Jane was a member of another of our kin groups – the Frosts (see Appendix A). She was in her early thirties when we interviewed her, and married with two young children. In total we interviewed six people from this kin group, including Jane's parents, Francis and June, and her two brothers: Andrew Frost, in his twenties and married, and Jack Frost, in his mid-thirties and married with a baby. The example we want to use is the relationships that Jane, and her brothers, have with their parents.

Our Frost interviewees gave us various examples of assistance passing between members of their kin group, but the most prominent channel of support was between Jane and her mother, June. June – who has her own investment income – regularly helped Jane financially, and also with various forms of practical support. Jane, for her part, gave her mother, and to a slightly lesser extent her father, practical help when needed. In fact, Jane's parents had not needed much help, except for a short spell when they were both (coincidentally) in hospital at the same time, but Jane has frequent contact with them – by telephone, and visiting. Jane characterised her relationship with her mother in particular as very close.

Jane's brothers, Andrew and Jack, have been less involved with their parents, in terms of emotional closeness, contact and regular practical support. When Francis and June were both hospitalised, Jane was to the fore in helping them on a daily basis, although Jack did also get involved. June explained it like this:

> *June*   There was an occasion when we were both in hospital together, and then I was in a month all told [which was longer than Francis]. And he [Francis] is absolutely hopeless at looking after himself, absolutely hopeless. And Jane was coming over two or three times a week, bringing cake and food and things for him, coming to see me, and bringing Rosie [Jane's daughter] with her. And you know, looking after him, doing his washing, doing my washing.

Should Francis and June need practical support or personal care at any stage in the future, it seems generally agreed among our interviewees that Jane will be the key provider of help.

How far does the idea of legitimate excuses shed light on the negotiation of support between parents and adult children in this kin group? We can identify both themes outlined above: the making of different excuses by men and women, and the making of the same kinds of excuses but under different conditions.

For example, employment is an area which differentiates Jane from her brothers in terms of excuses. The two Frost sons have 'done well' in their occupations – one as an accountant, one as a company secretary – and the demands of their employment are seen as an important priority in the family as a whole. Jane, who was a teacher but is now unemployed/looking after her young children, obviously sees her brothers as less available than herself if her parents need help. This is a view which her parents and brothers clearly share. For example, Andrew told us:

Andrew   When my parents have been unwell, you know, they've just, things have got to go on so er [pause] especially my sister I suppose because she's nearest and, maybe has more time because not being, not working, she helps out.

The point is that Jane does not have the excuse of employment in her repertoire, and although at some stage in the future she may return to employment, she is unlikely to achieve the high professional status of her brothers, in the eyes of the rest of her family. Although the Frosts are a 'middle-class' family, this distinction in employment status – in particular to accommodate child care – is common in our data set, as it is in national survey statistics (Martin and Roberts, 1984; Finch and Mason, 1990d).

Another area in which the biographies of Jane Smith and her brothers help to give them access to a different repertoire of excuses concerns questions of competence and skill. There seemed little doubt in the minds of our Frost interviewees that Jane was better than her brothers at certain domestic and caring tasks. For example, June explained what happened following her hospitalisation:

June   When I did come out of hospital Jack did come up two weekends and look after us over the weekends, you know, cook for us and everything. You know, they have given a lot of support. . . . But, er, yes Jane's very good, if I'm not well, she'll always come and look after me.
Interviewer   In what way do you think she is, I mean, you said earlier she's more caring than the other two, in what way is that so?
June   She seems to *know* what wants doing, and do it. I mean Jack would come over and cook a meal and bring the food with him. But he hasn't much sense of reality as to what sort of meal you want [laugh]. He fancies himself as a cook, I mean, he came over and brought a huge joint of meat, you know, a big joint of beef and things to cook it with, all the trimmings and things. Well, when you've not been very well that isn't what you want. What do you do with all the meat that's left? You know, and sort of not thinking. Whereas Jane would think what you'd like, and she's perhaps taken more note over the years as to the sort of things I would eat and like. [Emphasis in original]

It is perhaps not surprising that Jane is better at this kind of caring work, because her life experiences have allowed her to develop the necessary skills. But it does mean that it would be very difficult for Jane to argue that she was unable to provide practical or personal support because of a lack of competence. The process is therefore likely to be cumulative: Jane's caring skills, among other things, help to involve her in sets of developing commitments through which she increasingly builds up those kinds of skills.

There is a parallel here with our earlier comments about gender and skill, and the examples we used there, especially the Arkrights.

As well as showing that men and women can develop access to a different repertoire of excuses, the Frost example also helps to illustrate the operation of what seem to be similar excuses, but under different conditions for men and women. For example, aside from not having a job, a reason put forward as to why Jane had given most help to June and Francis when needed, and built up over time a more regularly supportive relationship with them, was that it was easier for her to get there because she did not live so far away. In fact, Jack lived about 160 miles away, Andrew about 60 miles, and Jane herself lived 40 miles away. While it is true that Jane lived the nearest, it is also the case that she did not actually live locally. It is not clear on the face of it why geography should not have functioned as a legitimate excuse for her too. In fact, it is only when geographical distance is seen in the context of the rest of her life, as compared to her brothers, that it starts to make sense as an excuse for them and not for her. It is significant that employment and geography, and their relative legitimacies, were tied up together here. For example, for the sons it was seen as an inevitable part of their careers that they might live at a distance from their parents. Furthermore, Andrew saw geographical distance from his parents as an important part of his claim to independence from them, and implicitly perhaps as a way of avoiding extensive commitments to assist kin. Jane had not seen distance from parents as an inevitable part of a career plan, and decisions about how near or far to live from them had very clearly been informed by the demands of the commitments which were developing between them. Jane was tending to treat responsibilities to kin as prior, and seeing distance as a barrier to be overcome. She was not even trying to use geography as an excuse. For her brothers it seems to have been treated more straightforwardly as preventing them from taking on commitments to their kin.

Understanding geographical distance in this kin group involves recognising that it is seen to mean something different in the context of different biographies and life experiences. Similar points can be made about how far commitments to 'one's own family' represent potentially the same excuse for men and women, but can actually mean very different things in practice. For Jane Smith, there is little doubt that the fact that she was looking after two young children at home made her look more rather than less available to take on regular practical and personal support of her parents. We saw this too in the Mansfield example earlier in this chapter, and in the case of Eileen Simpson in Chapter 3. Yet Jane Smith was seen in this way despite the fact that she lived 40 miles away from her parents, and her youngest child had an illness which demanded a great deal of care and attention. For her brothers, Jack and Andrew, the birth of a baby on the one hand, and the illness of his wife on the other, were both put forward as reasons why they were unable either to help their parents at particular times, or maintain such regular contact with them. For example, when June and Francis were in hospital:

> *June*   Poor Andrew, he'd got his wife in hospital with meningitis at the same time. So he couldn't do a thing, you know, he couldn't do anything but . . .
> *Interviewer*   No, he had to stay at home?
> *June*   I mean, she was more important, I mean there was nobody to look after her.

Some members of Andrew's wife's family of origin did come to stay and help during that period, but the point really is that June sees it as entirely legitimate that Andrew should prioritise his wife over his parents in this situation, rather than attempt to help all of them simultaneously.

We think we are picking up on a distinction here which is reflected in our data set as a whole: between the commitments of women who are looking after young children at home (generally not seen as a legitimate excuse for support which can in some senses complement it, even though that might be very difficult in practice), and other forms of commitment to one's 'immediate' family. It certainly seems to be the case that you can be more legitimately excused from fulfilling a commitment to a relative if you can claim successfully that it would mean putting that before the needs of your 'own family' (which is *not* the same as saying that there is a straightforward set of genealogical priorities). But gendered biographies can mean that women – unlike men – are seen as being in a position which makes them able to juggle various commitments simultaneously without the need to prioritise one over another. This is partly because women with young children at home are thought to live in conditions conducive to taking on other commitments (whether or not they really do), and also because those conditions are thought to help to generate the *skills* needed to juggle commitments.

As a result of these kinds of processes, women like Jane Smith do not have easy access to a range of excuses which they can successfully deploy in negotiations to claim that they are unable to help. In a situation like this one, where Jane's brothers *do* appear to have legitimate excuses, it is unsurprising that Jane and her family begin to view this particular developing commitment as her own personal responsibility.

There is a final point to make which applies not only to the Frosts, but more generally in our data set. Put quite simply, people are not always equally concerned with *trying* to get excuses accepted. For example, we noted earlier that Jane Smith did not really ever try to get her geographical distance from her parents accepted as an excuse for not helping them. Our understanding of Jane's behaviour here probably depends less on examining her repertoire of excuses *vis-à-vis* those of her kin, and more on the contours of her involvement in this particular commitment. In other words, by the time this particular need arose, Jane was not really in the business of trying to get excuses accepted as legitimate. In more general terms, this relates to our argument in Chapter 3 that women's biographies tend to put them in a position where they are particularly likely to develop commitments to relatives, and as a consequence to be regarded as an 'obvious' carer *without need for discussion*. Although we are not arguing that excuses are always made explicitly in discussions, the allocation of responsibility via a process of non-decision-making is often achieved without the person who ends up taking responsibility having tried to get excuses accepted as legitimate.

In conclusion to this section, we think that there is no straightforward relationship between gender and the ability to get an excuse accepted as legitimate, but there *is* a relationship. The arguments concerning genealogy are similar. In both cases, it is much more to do with understanding how commitments and reputations developed over time, and how women and men, or different categories of kin, are likely to be differentially positioned in this process. Their positioning is not *determined* by gender or genealogy, although it is influenced by them. What really matters is the influence of *this positioning* in relation to individual commitments in one's own family (not gender or genealogy *per se*), on one's opportunity to deploy and claim meanings in negotiations.

Does legitimacy matter?

The final question we are going to consider is whether or not it really matters that an excuse is accepted as legitimate. We think the answer to this question is yes it does matter, because there is a strong message in our data that people do seem to want their relatives to accept their excuses as legitimate. Although people sometimes fail in this, or are only partially successful, we cannot find any examples where people seem happy to have their relatives interpret their actions as illegitimate. It is also true that people may want their relatives' excuses to be legitimate. For example, we saw that Thomas MacIntyre wanted his father to be *legitimately* unable to help him and his siblings.

Asking whether legitimacy matters throws the focus very much on to the *moral* aspects of negotiations and responsibilities. For example, how far does an excuse need to have the moral approval of others in order to 'work'? Or to put in another way, what relationship does legitimacy have to whether or not an excuse works? If you end up not providing help, does it really matter if your position is not accepted as a legitimate one? This is another way of looking at whether or not legitimacy matters, and we think in practice there are at least three ways in which legitimacy and efficacy may be related. First, your excuse may be said to work if the result is that you do not provide the help in question, *and* everyone involved accepts this as a legitimate position. There are two different levels of efficacy involved here: whether or not you actually provide the help (if not, your excuse works at this level), and whether or not your position is accepted as legitimate (if so, your excuse works at this level). This combination represents the best possible form of excuse.

The second possibility is that no one accepts your position as legitimate, but you still do not provide support. In this version, the excuse is only working at one level, although people may try to persuade you to help even though they cannot *make* you do so. Our data suggest that people view this as the worst possible way of avoiding responsibilities, because they strive to have their actions seen in a different light.

The third variation is that you do not provide help, and your excuse is only partly accepted as legitimate, either because people are not wholly convinced, or because some are and others are not. Again, this form of excuse only works at one level, although the partial acceptance of legitimacy may mean that people do not actively put pressure on you to help.

In practice, what happens is often a combination of these variations, or aspects of them. Legitimacy matters, it seems, because without it people may run a number of risks. For example, if relatives perceive your position to be illegitimate they may actually put pressure on you to help. We saw this in the Mansfield example, where the sibling group successfully pressurised their mother to look after her estranged husband.

Another risk is that using illegitimate excuses may jeopardise your reputation, or personal identity, in your kin group. You may come to be known as someone who wilfully avoids responsibilities to kin. The effects of this may be quite pervasive and difficult to assess in advance, and we deal fully with this kind of question in the following chapter. Certainly though, as we have shown, having a reputation as someone who avoids responsibilities is not only an outcome of making excuses which are seen to be illegitimate, but also a factor which makes it more likely that excuses will be interpreted in that way in future.

A final example, which helps to bring out some of these points in a strong way, comes from Susan Mansfield's account of her father's response to the illness and eventual death of her mother. Susan, aged 39 when we interviewed her, begins her story by explaining why she did not go to school after the age of 14:

Susan My mother was ill, she was at home and I had two younger brothers and my father was working, so I was more or less off school to look after my mum until they took her to hospital. And after that I never went back, but they did know all about it.

Interviewer That must have been quite difficult for you at that age?

Susan That was terrible because, um up until then I was the only girl to my dad, he was my hero, you know, and at the time my mother, well she got cancer and um, he took it badly. When I say he took, I didn't realise at the time but he couldn't cope and of course he didn't come home you know, he'd stay out and then come home later on and, er that had a very bad effect on me. And for many years after I couldn't, I couldn't understand why, why he could do that, because to me, it wasn't for me and my brothers it was for my mum. You know, I mean, now I'm older, it must be terrible to be in that position. What would *I* do if somebody said how would *I* cope, would I run away from it, what would I do? I don't know. . . . Oh it was strange really, as I say, my Dad, she'd been ill two years earlier, she'd been in hospital, had an operation, and my Dad told me what was wrong with her. I would only be about 12 at the time. Thinking that I've always been sort of steady I suppose, he thought well I could cope [laugh], and I couldn't. But he couldn't cope either so, from then on she got better, and then she went back into decline. And he never [pause] he never, the thing that hurt was he never had a day off work to look after her. And as, I mean, it sort of sounds awful, but I was only a child and I thought that was wicked to do that, and I used to say to him well 'What's going to happen you know, what's going to happen?' 'Don't worry, I'll look after you', but it wasn't me I was asking for, and he didn't understand. [Emphasis in original]

Legitimacy matters terribly in this account. We cannot know how Susan's mother interpreted the situation, but we can surmise that for Susan's father the legitimacy of his own position mattered. By Susan's account he risked his continuing relationships with his family in general, and Susan in particular. One imagines it probably mattered very much to him personally, in terms of his own morality and personal identity. And it matters to Susan, who told us that although she can now understand her father's actions, she could not forgive him in his life-time, and still cannot after his death. She desperately wanted to be able to believe his excuses had been legitimate.

CONCLUSION

In this chapter we have begun to move the focus more directly on to aspects of negotiations between kin which are to do with the construction of meanings, and the interpretation of explanations and actions. We have used the concept of legitimate excuses to try to understand one dimension of this, and have focused both on the range of excuses we found in our data set, and the processes through which people try to get them accepted by their relatives as legitimate. We have argued that the ability to get an excuse accepted as legitimate is not just a straightforward product of *who* a person is (in terms of their gender or genealogical relationship to others involved), nor of *what* the excuse is.

Our exploration of the process of constructing an excuse, and getting it accepted, has led us to open up questions about the 'moral' aspects of negotiations between kin. In particular, we have suggested that moral reputations and identities are implicated in the process of constructing legitimacy. In the following chapter we turn the focus directly on to these moral aspects, and develop our analysis of their role in the negotiation of responsibilities between kin.

5 Reputations and moral identities in the negotiation of family responsibilities

INTRODUCTION: THE MORAL DIMENSIONS OF RESPONSIBILITIES TO KIN

In this chapter we will turn the spotlight explicitly on to what we are calling the 'moral dimensions' of negotiations about responsibilities in families. The importance of the moral dimension comes through in earlier chapters. For example, in Chapter 2 in our discussion of the balance between dependence and independence, it was clear there that people are not simply negotiating about the relative 'price' of the goods and services which they exchange, as weighed in material terms. In that sense the material value of the exchange is only one part of the picture. People are also negotiating about the boundaries of their relationships and about people's personal identities as 'dependent' or 'independent'. In Chapter 3, we noted the importance of 'moral and material baggage' which gets carried forward and reshaped through sequences of negotiations about support between kin. And in Chapter 4, we emphasised the relationship between the making of legitimate excuses and the construction of moral identities or reputations in kin groups. We are using the term 'moral dimensions' to cover these important facets of family responsibilities and the processes through which they are negotiated. We should underline that we do *not* mean 'moral rules' about responsibilities, but are using the term to refer to the non-material aspects of negotiations.

In focusing on the moral dimensions of relationships between kin, we are emphasing the 'how' rather than the 'what' of family life. We are suggesting that *the way* in which one individual interacts with another is just as important – and can be more important – than the substance of the goods and services which they exchange. Thus people try to present their actions in 'a good light'. We have seen this in previous chapters, both in our discussion of negotiating processes in Chapter 3 and in our discussion of legitimate excuses in Chapter 4. We are going to argue now that having one's actions seen in a good light is of general relevance for understanding relationships within kin groups. The way in which you conduct yourself in any negotiation with relatives can be taken to say something about you as a person. It can be remembered and used in the future – quite possibly long after the value of the goods and services exchanged has ceased to have any significance.

In talking about 'the how' of negotiations with relatives, we find it useful to employ the concept of demeanour, drawing on the work of Goffman (1967). Goffman uses the term to refer to the way in which a person conducts him or herself in face-to-face interactions. He argues that gestures, bearing and words all serve to convey a message that this person possesses certain attributes or qualities. The examples which he uses are qualities such as self-control, modesty and sincerity. We are more concerned with different qualities and attributes such as independence, reliability and generosity – but the argument still holds. No one can successfully establish that they possess these attributes simply by claiming that they do. It requires also that other people accept these claims *in practice*. This means that, in the course of social interactions, people make interpretations of how an individual handles him or herself, and attribute to that individual certain qualities on the basis of those interpretations. As Goffman summarises it, using only the male pronoun but presumably intending to include women as well as men in his analysis, 'Through demeanour an individual creates an image of himself, but properly speaking this is not an image that is meant for his own eyes' (1967: 78). The concept of demeanour, understood in this way, shows why it is important to look at the ways in which people conduct themselves, and also emphasises that we are not simply talking about matters of surface etiquette. In focusing on issues of demeanour we are making visible the means through which the moral identities of individuals are constructed.

As a preliminary example of what we mean, the case of Jane Jones highlights a number of important features. Jane was an elderly woman, one of the Jones kin group (see Appendix A) and the mother-in-law of Isobel Jones who was our initial contact in that family. Jane talked about the fact that she had lent £350 to her younger son (not Isobel's husband, who was dead) and had never been repaid despite having explicitly given the money as a loan.

> *Jane*   He came and he wanted to borrow money. And I'm a bit wary because he's a different type to my eldest son, he's a bit dodgy. So I says,'Have you spent that money I gave you, that £350?' 'No, no.' But I think it would have gone definitely. So I says,'Well I'll lend you another £350 but I want it back' [pause]. I'm still waiting. It's never been mentioned and *I* won't mention it. [Emphasis in original]

Other relatives had urged her to ask him for the money but she said that she would not do so. Her comment was, 'I wouldn't lower myself, that's just the difference you see.'

In this example we see that the key to understanding Jane's behaviour is demeanour. Indeed if we look just at her material interests in this situation her behaviour is puzzling. Why doesn't she ask for the money back? After all she made it clear before she gave it that it was a loan not a gift, and her son apparently agreed to this. The reason, as she presents it, is that it would reflect badly on herself. Her use of the phrase 'I wouldn't lower myself' carries a powerful message in this context. Despite the fact that, in the eyes of other people, she was a victim of her son's selfishness and completely entitled get her money back, actually to ask for something from a relative would have significantly damaged her moral identity. We also see that other members of the kin group form an audience for these transactions – it is not just a private matter between Jane and her son. She talks with other relatives about it, and they observe what she actually does. Both her son's reputation and hers are at stake.

Lying behind this issue specifically concerned with the loan, and complicating the transactions further, is the fact that Jane is the mother of the person she is criticising. Though we have quoted examples in other chapters (and we shall give more in this chapter) of people who make it pretty clear that they do not really like one of their parents, or a sibling, or some other relative, we have no direct examples in our data set of someone saying that they dislike one of their children. Jane Jones, in the incident which we have quoted, in fact is the person who comes the nearest to it. But elsewhere in her interviews she makes it clear that she is fond of him, appreciates his contact with her and still would be prepared to help him in other ways. Her feelings towards him no doubt are complex and categorising them as like or dislike is far too crude. But that is not our main point. What is striking is that neither she – nor any other parent – *portrays herself* as disliking a child. This in itself reinforces our point about demeanour. There is a sense in which for a parent (perhaps particularly a mother) to show that her overall feeling is dislike would reflect badly upon herself, as the person who brought up that child.

These points which we have drawn out of the Jane Jones example are ones which we will develop in the course of this chapter: the importance of demeanour; the ways in which moral identities are at stake; the kin group as 'audience' for negotiations between individuals. In the second half of the chapter we bring these themes together through an exploration of the concept of reputation as it applies to the negotiation of kin responsibilities.

ASKING AND OFFERING

We begin with a feature which is well recognised as part of the process of negotiating assistance within families: asking and offering. Do you ask for the help which you need, or do you wait for it to be offered? The distinction turns on whether the initiative is taken by the potential recipient or the potential donor. On first view this may seem very much a matter of surface etiquette, but in fact people commonly act as if much more is at stake, as is apparent in the case of Jane Jones.

From the Jane Jones case we might expect to find that the principle of 'not asking' is the dominant one. Indeed we do have many other cases in our interview data which demonstrate that this is important in the way that people conduct their relationships in practice. Nevertheless we have others which imply a more complex message. However, we will look first at our survey data, where we included several questions which enable us to probe asking and offering directly at the level of publicly expressed norms. The most elaborate of these is one of our longer vignettes concerning a man called John Highfield. The vignette concerns John's relationship with his parents over a financial matter. As part of this vignette, we built in questions which would distinguish between asking and offering. The relevant parts of the question read like this:

> John Highfield is a married man in his early thirties. He has a wife and two young children. John is unemployed but has a chance to start his own business. He can get various grants to help him get started, and the bank will lend most of the money he needs. But he still needs about £1500.
> a. If he thought his parents could afford to help, should he ask them for the money?
> b. (If yes) Should he ask for a gift or a loan?
> c. He does not like to ask his parents for the money, but should they *offer* it?

In response to the first part of this question, there is clear agreement among our survey respondents that John Highfield *should* ask his parents to help him financially: 88 per cent said that he should and only 8 per cent said that he should not (consensus baseline 75 per cent on this part of the question). In their responses to this question our survey respondents are clearly approving of someone asking a relative for help. However, we need to look beyond this.

In order to decide how to interpret this response we can compare it with another question, in which the principle of asking is not endorsed. This was a question about an elderly couple who need some money to redecorate their home (see Appendix B). Initially we asked whether relatives should *offer* money and we obtained a split pattern of answers, with 55 per cent saying that they should and 35 per cent that they should not (consensus baseline 75 per cent). To probe the issue of whether *asking* for help is appropriate in these circumstances, we asked those 342 respondents who had said that relatives should 'not offer' whether the elderly couple should *ask* relatives for help and 70 per cent said that they should not, with 20 per cent saying that they should. This does not quite reach our consensus baseline of 75 per cent, but contrasts sharply with the pattern of answers to the John Highfield question.

What are the features of these two questions which might account for the different messages about 'asking'? First there are differences in the circumstances of the people needing help. The circumstances of John Highfield's situation were particularly conducive to the response that he should receive assistance. He was a good 'deserving case' – a man with a young family, doing his best to establish himself economically. As we indicated in Chapter 1, in general our survey population were most inclined to approve of assistance from relatives where they were deserving cases, of which this is one. Also we proposed that the help might come from his parents specifically. Again we noted in Chapter 1 that parents' continuing assistance towards their children is the situation in which people are most likely to endorse help from relatives. By contrast, in the case of the elderly couple needing money for decorating, the help would have to pass from the younger to the older generation and, in addition, their need may have been perceived as less urgent and therefore their circumstances as less deserving. Also we should note that the respondents who answered the question about whether the elderly couple 'should ask' were the group least favourable to the idea of the help coming from relatives.

So it is understandable that our survey respondents approved of John's parents assisting him financially. But are they straightforwardly endorsing the principle of *asking*? Are they saying that, provided the case is a deserving one and that relatives are the most suitable source of help, it is perfectly acceptable for the potential recipient to take the initiative? We think that it is a bit more complex than this. In the second part of the John Highfield question we asked the 862 respondents who said that John *should* ask his parents for financial help whether he should ask for a gift or a loan and 98 per cent said a loan. This is the highest level of agreement for any question in our survey and easily exceeds our consensus baseline of 75 per cent. It suggests that, when people said that John should ask his parents for money, they also had in mind that he should do this in a particular kind of way. It is acceptable for him to take the initiative and ask, but what he should be asking for is a loan not a gift. In a sense this reinforces the point about deservingness. In asking for a loan not a gift, John would be showing that he was not seeking to become 'too dependent' on his parents (see Chapter 2). But also, asking for a loan implies that his parents can retain some control over the situation by setting the terms, and that ultimately they will not be financially disadvantaged.

The implication of this vignette is that people do not consider that asking for help is unacceptable in all circumstances. Indeed in some circumstances it may be very appropriate. What matters is *what* you are asking for and *how* you ask. It is clear that John should *not* ask for a gift. At the same time evidence from the vignette also supports the view that being in a position where you 'have to ask' is undesirable and that, in such a situation, the potential donor has some responsibility to avert the difficulties by taking the initiative to make an offer.

We get this from the third part of the vignette, where we posed the problem that John might not like to ask his parents, especially if he thought that lending him money would cause them some financial hardship. In these circumstances there was a notable measure of agreement among our respondents that the parents have a responsibility to offer the assistance needed: 78 per cent said that they should offer and 11 per cent said that they should not (consensus baseline 75 per cent). The same applies in another of our shorter survey questions, about a 19-year-old woman with a baby, where the issue is whether she should return to her parents' home to live (see Chapter 1 and Appendix B). Our respondents strongly favoured her going back to her parents' home: 79 per cent said that she should and 14 per cent said that she should not (consensus baseline 75 per cent). Given that this is another question about parents helping a young adult child, it is not surprising that our survey population favours help being given. However, as with the question about the elderly couple needing money to decorate their home, we then asked those who said she should *not* go back whether the parents should *offer* their daughter a home. There were 200 people in this group and 77 per cent of them said yes (consensus baseline 75 per cent). Thus even where respondents thought that parental support was not a desirable outcome, they still felt that the parents had a responsibility to offer it.

This endorsement of the donor's 'responsibility to offer' underlines our basic point that, at the level of publicly expressed norms as well as in practice, it is definitely preferable for a potential donor to take the initiative. A donor sensitive to the moral as well as the material dimensions of these exchanges should ensure that an offer is made before the prospective recipient is placed in a position where he or she 'has to ask'. If she has to ask, it is difficult for her actions to be cast in a good light, and her moral identity is thus at risk. This was the main thing which Jane Jones held against her son (in the example discussed earlier in this chapter). It was not so much that he had broken his promise to repay the money lent by his mother. It was that he had put her moral identity at risk by placing her in a position where she 'had to ask' him to repay.

We will explore the dynamics of asking/not asking in practice by discussing whether and how these principles are reflected in the rest of our interview data. But before we do that, we need to introduce a related principle: 'expecting' or 'not expecting' to receive help.

NOT EXPECTING

In a straightforward sense 'expecting' help is different from 'asking' for it because expecting refers to the way someone *thinks* about the possibility of getting support, while asking refers to what he or she *does* about this possibility. We shall argue that in reality the two overlap, but initially in our analysis we will maintain the distinction between them and focus on the issue of 'expecting'.

There is a certain logic in the view that a responsibility to give help does imply a corresponding right to expect it. However, this view is not reflected in our data. Indeed we get strong messages that the majority of our respondents see it as *wrong* to expect assistance from relatives in time of need, even to expect recompense for assistance given previously, in the sense of *assuming* it will automatically be given. These messages come from both our survey and our interview data. It seems to be the idea of 'expecting' which lies at the heart of this, and which people reject.

We will look first at our survey data, where we asked some questions which were concerned with expecting recompense for assistance given to a relative. We can see that people reject the idea of 'expecting', at the level of publicly expressed norms about family life. The most straightforward survey question which addresses this issue runs like this:

> Should a person who is caring for a sick or elderly relative expect to get something, however small, from that relative in return, or should relatives expect to give their time for nothing?

Of our respondents 83 per cent said that a person should expect to give their time for nothing and only 13 per cent said that they should expect something in return (consensus baseline 75 per cent). In interpreting the answers to this question, we need to consider whether respondents were disapproving principally of the idea that someone should *expect* to receive a reward, rather than of the idea that recompense *itself* is inappropriate. The wording of this question runs the two issues together. It may well be that the strength of the response to this question turns on the idea that someone should *expect* to get something in return when they do a favour for a relative, though simply on the basis of answers to this question we cannot be sure.

The same issue arises in one of our longer vignettes, where we can take our interpretation a bit further. The story told in this vignette concerns a mother, daughter and grand-daughter and the question of what responsibilities they should acknowledge to each other, in the context of the particular set of relationships which they have built up over time. We are concentrating here mainly on the relationship between mother and daughter. (We have discussed the relationship between grandmother and grand-daughter in Chapters 2 and 4, and also in Finch and Mason, 1990d.) The wording for the relevant part of this vignette is as follows:

> This situation is about Mary Harper, an elderly woman who has one widowed daughter, Valerie. She has quarrelled with Valerie and cut her out of her will. So Valerie knows that she will not inherit her mother's house. Her mother is too frail to live alone any more and does not want to go into a home. The daughter, Valerie, is not sure what to do. On the one hand she has enough space for her mother. On the other hand they have never got on well together.
> a. What should Valerie do?
>   Offer her mother a home.
>   Arrange for her mother to go into a nursing home.
>   Something else (specify).
> b. If Valerie *did* offer her mother a home would it be reasonable to say that her mother must change her will and leave the house; or should Valerie offer her mother a home without any conditions?

On the main question of whether Valerie *should* offer her elderly mother a home despite the history of their very poor relationship, our respondents are divided: 37 per cent say that she should offer her mother a home and 51 per cent say that she should arrange for her mother to go into a nursing home. Neither of these responses reaches our consensus baseline of 75 per cent. However, on the second part of the question the pattern is much clearer and reflects the answers given to our other question on expecting recompense: 82 per cent of our respondents said that, if Valerie did offer her mother a home, that offer should be made without any conditions; only 13 per cent said that Valerie should ask her mother to change her will (consensus baseline 75 per cent).

Although this is not surprising in the light of our other question about expecting recompense, it underlines the clarity of the message that, for most people, it is wrong even under the most trying of circumstances to make explicit that you expect a relative to repay the help that you are giving to them. In this vignette the daughter has a longstanding poor relationship with her mother. Her mother has expressed her negative view of her only daughter by taking the rather unusual step of excluding her from her will. Valerie nonetheless is still prepared to contemplate taking her mother to live with her in her old age. Yet our respondents seem to be saying that, even in *these* circumstances, she should not take the initiative to ensure that her apparently rather generous actions get rewarded in some way.

The responses to the vignette are capable of two possible interpretations. One is that respondents reject the whole idea of 'expecting', implying that the idea of recompense should not even enter Valerie's head. The other is that what is inside Valerie's head is not really the issue. Respondents' disapproval is actually focused on the fact that Valerie acts in a way which implies that she expects something in return. To put it in Goffman's language, her demeanour conveys the message that she expects recompense, and this is the important factor in shaping our respondents' judgements. It is at this point that we begin to see the overlap between expecting help and asking for help. The two are linked through the concept of demeanour. We would suggest that our data on asking and offering need to be seen in this light. It is not so much that asking as such is disapproved of. It is what asking *implies*. If someone asks for help there is a danger that other people will perceive their actions as implying that they expect to receive it. And – at least at the level of publicly endorsed beliefs – 'expecting' is strongly rejected. Thus from this vignette question we would conclude that, at the level of what would be endorsed publicly as the proper way to behave, most people say that it is wrong to *act as if* you expect repayment.

If these interpretations which focus on demeanour are correct, this suggests that it is more important to know how a person's actions are presented to and interpreted by other people, than it is to try to understand what they 'really expect', or perhaps more generally what they 'really think'. Our survey data can take us no further than hinting at the importance of this. Our interview data enable us to explore more about the process of negotiating, and how far these principles are reflected in our interviewees' own experiences and in their thinking about relationships with their own kin.

In our interview data, we can identify some examples where it is implied that expecting help from relatives *is* acceptable, and others where it is not. We will consider these in turn. In total we have identified forty-four examples where an interviewee is telling us that showing you expect help *is* acceptable. Usually this also involves taking the initiative to ask for it. Most examples concern incidents which have happened in the past, but some refer to an interviewee's view of what they would do in the future if they needed a particular type of help. About one third of these examples, where asking seems acceptable, are about young adults asking for help from parents (or in one or two cases, another older relative). This is consistent with the pattern which we have identifed elsewhere, and which suggests that help from parents to children in adult life is regarded differently from other types of assistance in families. Our data on 'asking' suggest that children can ask their parents for help in ways which do not apply in other relationships.

In our other examples, it seems that there are circumstances which *may* make asking acceptable, for instance if the assistance would clearly be part of a reciprocal exchange. A typical example of this would be Jean Crabtree, talking about what she does when she needs emotional or moral support:

> *Jean*   Emotional support – I would say, yes. We talk our problems out among each other. You know, perhaps I'll go and see my sister and talk to my mum – and vice versa. We do usually talk a lot, if we have a problem. I'd, you know, go and see one of them.

Jean is saying that she is quite happy to approach her mother or her sister if she needs to talk over a problem because she knows that they will come to her when they need the same sort of help. 'Asking' does not, in a case like this, disturb the dependence–independence balance. In a sense the underlying logic here is rather like John Highfield asking for a loan: it implies that there will not be a net gain for the person who asks. In fact several examples from our interview data where asking was acceptable *did* entail asking for loans. This lends weight to our argument that one circumstance in which asking may be acceptable is where ultimately there will be no net material gain, and where the balance of dependence and independence will be undisturbed in the long run.

These kinds of examples are rather far removed from the idea of a 'right to expect' help. We really have only one example in our data set where an interviewee makes it explicit that he sees himself as having the right to expect (almost to demand) assistance. This is the case of John Green and his relationship to his grandchildren, which we discussed in Chapter 2. John had helped his grandchildren financially in various ways and had made them beneficiaries in his will. He felt that therefore he did have a right to expect their practical assistance with tasks in the house and garden, now that he was getting older. He put it like this:

> *John*   That's the sort of help I would expect [pause]. And I would. I would *expect* to get it too. I wouldn't think they were doing me any favours because I've done the same things for them. I've helped them financially and I've done jobs, all that sort of thing. So I reckon I'm entitled to expect the same sort of assistance from them. [Emphasis in original]

We should emphasise that this is our only example which implies a strong concept of the 'right to expect' and which presents it, in effect, as a straightforward corollary of the 'obligation to give' assistance. In other examples in our interview data people explicitly reject the notion that there is anything approaching a right to expect, even between parents and children.

In total we have identified thirty-six examples which carry the message that expecting help is not acceptable. We shall use a detailed exploration of one of these examples as the framework for discussing this issue of not expecting.

We have chosen this example because it brings out the issue of demeanour explicitly. Interestingly it comes from our interview with Teresa Green, John's wife, though it involves a different aspect of their family relationships. It concerns their negotiations, at the time of their marriage ten years previously, around having Teresa's mother to live with them. She had previously shared a house with Teresa for many years. Teresa was in her early fifties when she married John. She had not been married previously and she worked in a professional, high-status job in the welfare field. John and Teresa both told us that they realised that the question of whether to offer a home to Teresa's mother had significant implications for them, and both were agreed that the decisive initiative had come from John. It is Teresa's account which we are going to quote here, because she recounts the process of making the decision in a way which emphasises the importance of *how* it was done.

> *Interviewer*   We are interested in who suggested what to who. Do you remember how it was actually . . .
> *Teresa*   How my mother came here?
> *Interviewer*   Well yes. How did it develop?
> *Teresa*   Well my husband suggested it. I wouldn't have because I don't think I have any right to suggest [pause]. I knew perfectly well that my mother would be totally dependent as soon as she stepped over this threshold [pause]. I wouldn't have suggested it, you know. And didn't in fact [pause].
> *Interviewer*   So then you put it to her did you?
> *Teresa*   Oh well, she was just waiting to be asked [pause]. In fact she hadn't thought there was an alternative solution, I don't think.

In Teresa's account both she and her mother apparently acted as if it would be wrong of them to expect an invitation for the latter to live with Teresa and John after their marriage. Both treated John as the person who had to take the initiative, the one who had the power ultimately to give or withhold the invitation, on the grounds that the implications were greatest for him, as the new husband. This has some parallels with the Simpson case (discussed in Chapter 3) where Stan wanted Eileen to approve actively of inviting his mother to live with them. In both cases the child-in-law is treated as someone who should properly be accorded the right of veto.

However, in the Green case, Teresa makes it clear that her mother actually *did* expect to move in with them ('she was just waiting to be asked. She hadn't thought that there was an alternative solution'). Though it is not entirely clear from what Teresa says, the implication is that her mother 'hinted' that she might come to live with them. In some other examples in our data set, hinting is a mechanism identified explicitly. For example Ann Jones and her brother Zaki, both young single adults, described how they had received various types of financial help from their mother and one grandmother through processes which seemed usually to entail hinting. Ann confirmed this when she described her family generally as 'great hinters'. Hinting is a process which enables someone to make their needs known, while at the same time preserving the principle that you should not ask for help directly, and not show that you expect to get it.

To return to Teresa Green, it seems that her mother *did* expect to move in with Teresa and John. But Teresa herself seems not actually to have envisaged an alternative either. On one level, the behaviour of the two women in this scenario seems to be a matter of etiquette – showing that they understand it is polite to wait to be asked. But at another level Teresa makes it clear that to have spoken or acted as if she expected her mother to live with them would have transgressed more than etiquette. She says, 'I don't think I have any right to suggest' and reinforces this by saying later 'I wouldn't have suggested it and I didn't in fact'.

Why does Teresa express herself strongly on the point that she had 'no right to suggest' her mother's living in her home? We will draw out three points here, each of which can be supported with other examples in our data set. First, we would argue that the reason why she had 'no right' to suggest this move is that she would have been claiming for herself the rights that all of them agreed implicitly should rest with her husband – the person whose life would be changed most significantly if her mother moved in with them, since Teresa and her mother had shared a home for many years. To make the suggestion that her mother should live with them after their marriage would put pressure on John and would have taken away his ability to offer assistance freely, or to decide to withhold it. We have several other examples which parallel this quite closely.

The principle which lies behind this can be expressed in general terms. Showing that you expect a favour is unacceptable because it alters the balance in a set of relationships. In particular it takes away some of the rights which should properly be left with the donor (defined as John Green, in this case). It is for this reason that the 'obligation to give' does *not* imply the 'right to expect'. It may well be that an endorsement of this principle lies behind the responses we got from our survey respondents to the Harper vignette, at least in part. In our qualitative data set, about one-third of the examples which indicate that expecting is wrong imply clearly this issue of taking away the donor's rights. One example is the case of Jane Smith, which we discussed in Chapter 2, who objected to her mother-in-law and her sister-in-law making demands on the use of her car. Very clearly in this case, Jane was not being left the freedom to take a decision about whether she would use her own resources to the benefit of relatives.

There are various mechanisms available which appear to get round this problem to an extent, and which get used in families. We have already noted that 'hinting' rather than asking is one. Another is asking for something less than you actually need, leaving the donor the flexibility of deciding whether to offer more. An example of this comes from Sara Anwar, a young woman of Asian descent who was living rent-free in her parent's house when we interviewed her. She and her young son had moved in when her husband went to work abroad. Sara described how she had offered to pay her mother rent, but the offer was refused. In asking for her parents to provide accommodation, but offering to pay them for it, she had been making a request which was less than she needed (because her salary as a community worker was low), but which left her parents in the position of taking the final decision about precisely what they would offer to her.

The second point which we want to draw from Teresa Green's comment that she had 'no right to suggest' is that it highlights the significance of demeanour. It is *showing* that you expect an offer to be made which puts on the pressure, not the private thoughts which you keep to yourself. Again this is reflected in other interviews in our qualitative data set – about one-third of our examples which emphasise 'not expecting' have this feature. For example Jean Crabtree, a woman in her early twenties, told us about the close relationship which she had with her mother Ellen and how, though Ellen was perfectly fit and healthy, Jean and her boyfriend frequently helped her with domestic tasks like decorating. However, Jean emphasised that the initiative never came from her mother, 'she wouldn't ask any of us to do it [pause]. She doesn't expect us to.' In formulating it this way, Jean implies that the key sign that her mother 'doesn't expect' is that she *wouldn't ask*. She reinforced this by linking it with her own future relationship with any children she might have, showing that she sees assistance from children to parents as something which should be experienced as given freely, rather than under pressure of 'being expected'.

> *Jean*   I wouldn't expect them to be always helping me [pause]. I don't think you bring children into the world for your own old age thinking, you know, they'll be able to come and help me [pause]. If they want to help you that's fine, but I wouldn't like to pressure anyone into helping me.

The idea of 'putting pressure' on the potential donor clarifies further why *asking* for help is problematic. Asking is suspect because it implies that you 'expect' help, we have already argued. We can now also see that anything which shows that you expect help – or perhaps more importantly is *perceived as showing* this – reflects badly on you because you seem to be usurping the right of the donor to offer or withhold assistance. It implies that you are the kind of person who does not respect the rights of others, selfishly attempting to let your own needs override these.

Third, the example of Teresa Green suggests that the process of 'showing that you expect' an offer of assistance not only affects the position of the donor, but also reflects badly upon yourself. When she says, 'I wouldn't have suggested it, and I didn't in fact' she is making claims about the kind of person she is – someone who would not act in this way. Her personal moral identity was bound up in the way in which this situation was handled, and she is telling us that she came out of it well. Similarly Jean Crabtree indicates that she does not wish to be seen as the kind of person who would 'pressure anyone into helping me'.

About two-thirds of our examples of 'not expecting' suggest that moral identity is implicated. Quite commonly, it is the identity of 'being independent' which, as we showed in Chapter 2, is an important consideration for both young and old. For example Alfred King, an elderly man living alone when we interviewed him, stressed that he had 'never asked' for help from his family, and linked that explicitly with the fact that he was 'very independent'. Similarly Sophia Ellis described her Asian grandparents as being unwilling to ask relatives for help because it would damage 'their own dignity and self-respect'. At the opposite end of the age range, Jim Turner, a man in his twenties with four children who had been unemployed for several years, told us that he tried hard to avoid asking relatives for help because 'the older you get the less you want to depend on anyone else'. In all these cases, the identity of each individual as an independent adult was bound up with 'not asking' and 'not expecting'. Other examples focus on different facets of identity, for example being unselfish or being generous (which we consider in the next section).

Before concluding our discussion of expecting and not expecting, we need to note a gender dimension to all this. The thirty-six examples which emphasise that it is wrong to expect assistance were given to us by twenty-six individuals, sixteen women and ten men. The forty-four examples which indicated that expecting is acceptable came from thirty-seven individuals, twelve women and fifteen men. Though the differences are not absolute, there is a varying gender balance in each set of examples. Men, who formed slightly less than half our study population (see Appendix A) gave us more examples than women of situations where it *is* acceptable to expect help from a relative. Women however were the larger group when it came to examples where the message was that expecting help is *not* acceptable. Numerically the differences are relatively small. But when we look at *what* people say about these issues, the people who talk most extensively about 'not expecting', and especially those who emphasise matters of demeanour, are all women. Our only example of a man who started to talk in these terms is interesting, because in a sense it reinforces our point about gender differences. Alf Smith made the following comments, while considering the issue of what would happen if his parents were to need substantial help in old age:

Interviewer So you know that they would expect you to help them?
Alf Well [pause] I wouldn't say *expect*. I don't know. I mean it's hard to define really isn't it? You say they don't expect it and yet if you don't offer it, they're going to be really hurt like. So really, deeper down, they must ruddy well expect it in the first place, you know [laughs].

Alf shows, in this extract, that he finds it difficult to disentangle the issue of what people 'really expect' from what they say, showing in effect that he does not have the same grasp of the complexities of these processes as do some of the women – for example Teresa Green or Jean Crabtree, whom we have quoted in this section.

In general the impression from our interview data is that women tend to be more finely attuned to these processes. Though obviously it is not possible for us to make broad generalisations about women and men on the basis of these data, it seems important to note this difference. Certainly one can suggest explanations of why it might be more important for women than for men to develop a finely tuned sense of the importance of 'not expecting' assistance from relatives. That explanation would centre on the different importance which relationships with relatives generally have for women and men, and on the greater likelihood that women will need to rely on kin for assistance at various points throughout their adult lives – therefore they *need* to bother more about the way in which their own reputations are constructed in the process of negotiating assistance.

In conclusion we would argue that this discussion of 'not expecting' shows the importance of demeanour – of the *way* in which negotiations between relatives are conducted – and indicates that its importance is linked to the construction of the moral identities of individuals. Demeanour is more than etiquette because it implies moral attributes and qualities. We have isolated the processes around asking, offering and expecting as a key to understanding the significance of this. Though there are circumstances in which asking for, and even expecting to receive, help is acceptable there is a strong theme in our data that the rights of the donor to offer or withhold assistance must be respected and protected. In turn it is reflected in a general wariness about asking for help. But that also leaves open the possibility that asking is perfectly acceptable, provided it can be done in a way which does not usurp the rights of the donor.

In a sense this underlines the points that we have made, in different ways, in earlier chapters, that family responsibilities are not a matter of fixed rules of obligation, attached to specific genealogical positions. Offering help to a relative is much more like a process of gift-giving. There is a small but interesting body of social science literature on gift-giving beginning with the classic work of Marcel Mauss (1954), which emphasises that giving gifts is not just an exchange of material commodities but is also a moral transaction, which creates and consolidates social relationships and moral obligations (see also Cheal, 1987, 1988; Corrigan, 1989). Our analysis of family responsibilities certainly fits with that view, as our discussion in Chapter 2 makes clear when we outline the importance of reciprocating. However, we would emphasise that we are talking about a gift-giving of a particular type, one which sees each individual potentially with a considerable degree of freedom to choose whether a gift will be given, and what type of gift it will be. In the next section we develop this notion of 'giving' in a different way by looking at the process of being generous.

BEING GENEROUS

The concept of generosity in family relationships in a sense is the polar opposite of 'expecting'. By definition generosity means that assistance is given well beyond anything which the recipient could have a 'right to expect'. It apparently represents a clear case where the donor is under no pressure from the expectations of the recipient. We are going to look at examples of generosity in our interview data, from the perspective of the key themes which we are developing in this chapter. In what circumstances do actions get defined as 'being generous'? What is the interplay between the moral and material dimensions of the interaction in these instances? How are moral identities implicated in such transactions? How important is it to conduct 'generous' transactions in the right way?

We have various cases in our data set where people told us about examples of assistance between kin which were defined as 'generosity'. On some occasions, these involved the kind of assistance which makes a very significant difference to the life of the person receiving it. We take a key example here from the Archer kin group (see Appendix A for details). It is the example in our interview data set which represents the largest single sum of money mentioned by any of our interviewees as a gift or loan between relatives. In that sense it is not typical. However, it does enable us to see very clearly some of the processes at work when a gift is defined as generous within families. Those same processes are reflected in other examples where the gift is less valuable in material terms, as we shall show.

We refer to the gift from John and Dorothy O'Malley of £10,000 (at

1970s prices) to Phil Archer their son-in-law, to enable him to buy a partnership in a veterinary practice. Though it would be possible for this to be treated as a business investment rather than a gift, all parties to the transaction (all of whom we interviewed) presented it as a gift from parents to children, an example of family assistance not of a business arrangement. The agreement was that the capital sum was to be treated as a gift, in effect as an advance on the parents' estate which would pass to their daughter Jill and her family in any case on the parents' death. However, Phil was to pay his parents-in-law the equivalent of the interest which they would have earned on this capital, as they relied on it to supplement their income in retirement. All the members of the family whom we interviewed cited this as an example of the kind of assistance which characterised their relationships, which were clearly very warm. Those at the receiving end presented it as a prime example of the parent's generosity, as is apparent in this extract from Jill's interview, 'My parents are *totally* generous. They even feel guilty about the interest that they take and we insist, we've had to twist their arm to take it.' The essence of this arrangement is that it was seen by the participants as going well beyond the types of exchanges which normally pass between parents and children. In that sense the whole point of it is that it is *not* characteristic of support within families. Yet in another sense it *is* an arrangement characteristic of family life. As John O'Malley put it, 'We wouldn't do it for anyone else. You wouldn't think about it. But you do it for your own.'

In commenting upon this as an example of generosity, we will make three points. First, on the surface it seems that this gift was characterised as 'generous' because it went well beyond what children have a 'right to expect'. However, in another sense it was tied into a set of expectations about how parents and children should behave towards each other, which everyone understood. It was seen as entirely *appropriate* that parents act in this way towards their children ('We wouldn't do it for anyone else but you do it for your own'). Being generous to your children is what parents do, yet if children *expect* their parents to make large gifts to them, this robs them of the right to have their actions defined as generosity. At the same time, it is this sense of appropriateness which made it possible for the children to accept the gift.

Second, it is clear in this example that demeanour is extremely important. The children's moral identities were at stake and it was important for them to show that they did 'not expect' the gift. When they get it, they must receive it in the right way. Dorothy O'Malley said that Jill and Phil had been 'very grateful' and John emphasised that they had paid back the interest 'regularly and religiously' despite the fact that they had been told that this did not really matter. To have acted in any other way of course would have called into question the definition of the gift as generous and would have turned it into something over which the children were claiming some rights. They needed to *go on* treating it as generous and to demonstrate this through their actions. The parents' moral identities as well as the children's were implicated here. Following Goffman's argument, we could say that they could only establish their identities as 'generous parents' if their children treated them as such.

Third, this example of being generous did have implications for the balance of the relationship between the generations. Until the money was repaid, Jill and Phil would always be the recipients of a gift which they had no right to expect. We can see here how being the donor of a generous gift can put you in a powerful position *vis-à-vis* the receiver of the gift. This is similar to Mauss's analysis of gift giving and suggests that there is a fine line between receiving a generous gift and becoming 'beholden to' the giver (Mauss, 1954). In Jill and Phil Archer's case, being beneficiaries of parents' generosity created a further set of responsibilities – at least of a generalised if not a direct kind. Jill Archer told us that she feels an impulse to be generous with financial assistance to her own children, linking this explicitly to the way in which her parents have treated her. Indeed we used Jill in Chapter 2 as one of our examples of indirect repayment across generations.

Thus acts of generosity both fall outside the normal scope of reciprocal responsibilities and also are part of them. They are part of them precisely because they are constructed in a way which makes them appear separate from any structure of obligation yet, at another level, they are a characteristic part of family life because you would 'do it for your own' but not for other people. The effect of the generous gift in the Archer family had not only been to assist Phil in his career but also to bind the family together in a different way, both financially and morally.

The recognition that generosity has this effect may perhaps lead people to reject generous gifts, or at least to try to repay them so that they then become part of the more usual process of exchange. One case where this apparently had happened is in the Jackson family (see Appendix A for details) where Robert, at an earlier stage in his life, had received money from his parents to cover his basic financial needs at a time when he was out of work. Robert described this to us as a generous gift, an example that showed how his parents 'were only too willing to give us every penny they had'. It was also clear that it was intended to be a gift not a loan: 'they did it without thought of repayment'. However, Robert felt that he did not want to accept money from his parents on these terms, describing himself as a person who will not accept anything without at least a verbal promise of repayment. As far as we can tell, the parents did not argue with him at that point. Presumably they accepted it as appropriate in the circumstances that Robert was promising to repay – a sign that Robert was treating the gift as something which he did not have the right to expect. However, when he was more financially secure, Robert not only wanted to pay back the amount which his parents had given, but also to give them substantially more, because he knew that they were dependent upon a small pension. By this action he was, in effect, reversing the balance of generosity. This was strongly resisted by Mary and Richard Jackson, as Robert describes:

> *Robert* It was a case of writing a cheque out and saying 'Thank you very much for everything. You've helped me so much.' My mother turned round and said 'Well you didn't borrow this off us. It wouldn't come to anywhere near this amount what we gave you – not lent you, but gave you.' And er, I mean she gave me the cheque back three times and said 'I don't want it.' And I said 'Well whether you want it or not, if you give me your bank book, I'll go and put it in myself.' And she was very reluctant to accept it.

The negotiations being conducted here are clearly about very much more than the need of the respective parties for money. At one level, they can be interpreted as an example of the processes which we discussed in Chapter 2 – restoring the dependence–independence balance between Robert and his parents. In accepting money from his mother and father to supply his basic needs and those of his household, Robert had called into question his own independence. In a sense he had put himself in a position where they had authority over him in a way more reminiscent of childhood than adulthood. Whether or not they chose to exercise this it was important for Robert to restore the balance, it can be argued.

But the issues also go beyond this. They touch upon the moral identities of both Robert and his parents, around the theme of generosity. Robert is establishing his own identity not only as someone who repays debts but also as someone who himself is generous to others. At the same time his actions call into question the definition of his parents' original gift as 'generous'. He is treating it as a loan to be paid back, not as a gift which stands outside the normal expectations of reciprocal responsibilities. Thus although we are told that in material terms the parents could certainly use the money (this is confirmed in various ways in interviews with this family) the moral dimensions weighed more heavily with Mary and she was 'very reluctant to accept it'. It is the importance of the moral dimension which gives Robert's account of this interaction with his mother something of a ritual flavour. It seems to have been important both for Robert to offer the money and also for Mary to resist it. The process of going through these negotiations may be more important in the end than whether any money actually changes hands, precisely because what they are really negotiating about is their respective moral identities. Having established herself firmly as someone who resists the repayment of generosity, Mary finally is able to accept money from her son.

Most examples of actions which our interviewees defined as 'generous' were on a much smaller scale than in the case of the Jacksons or the Archers. Indeed some of these instances involved fairly minor examples of assistance but these were important nonetheless in shaping the character of the relationship between the individuals involved. One such example comes from our interview with Ethel Phillips, a woman in her sixties and living alone but in fairly good health. Ethel described how her daughter-in-law took regular care of her welfare. She would often ring her at weekends and ask her down for tea so that Ethel would not have to be on her own; she frequently sent one of her children to their grandmother's house with small gifts for their grandmother (a pint of milk was given as an example); and she was in the habit of telephoning Ethel every night to make sure that she was alright. Ethel clearly saw this as going well beyond what one could expect a daughter-in-law to do, 'She's a good girl you know [pause]. I mean to say, there's not many daughters-in-law like that.' Although the word 'generosity' may imply gifts of money, the example of Ethel Phillips makes it clear that actions as well as goods can be defined as generous in families. They meet the criterion that the parties define them as going well beyond what anyone has a right to expect, and that they stand outside the normal expectations that a gift will be matched with a counter-gift. In Ethel Phillips' case, making daily telephone calls was a key element in the construction of her daughter-in-law as generous.

In conclusion, we would underline that actions which get defined as 'generous' on one level stand outside the normal processes of giving and receiving, of paying back, of balancing dependence and independence. At another level they are part of the same processes through which assistance gets negotiated in families. They have implications for the balance of relationships, and for the moral identities of all the parties, as well as possibly being valuable in material terms. Bringing together our discussion of 'expecting' and 'generosity', we would underline that the processes involved here are very complex to understand – far more complex than we see if we look only at the material dimensions of assistance within kin groups, and focus upon the objective value of the goods and services which are given. The interweaving of the material and the moral dimensions of exchanges comes through very clearly here and, in many instances, the moral seems more prominent than the material. It is far from easy to get your actions accepted and understood in a way which reflects well upon yourself. Yet at times people seem to treat this as more important than anything else. To understand more fully why this is so, we turn now to look at the concept of reputation within family relationships.

REPUTATION IN THE KIN GROUP

In this chapter we have discussed the 'moral identities' of individuals and we have argued that giving and receiving assistance in families involves not only the exchange of money, goods and services, but also negotiations about the identities of individuals. We shall go on now to develop this theme by linking this discussion of moral identities with the concept of 'reputation'. We shall argue that individuals do build up specific reputations within their families and that these are both a *product* of past negotiations with kin and a *component* of future negotiations. These ideas emerged in our discussions of negotiations in Chapter 3, and of legitimate excuses in Chapter 4. We are going to develop them fully here.

By introducing the concept of reputation at this point we want to emphasise the importance of looking at the way relationships develop over time. Reputations, we shall argue, are the means by which the moral identity of each individual gets built up, consolidated and modified over time, and gets 'carried' from one situation to another. Given that our focus is centrally on processes within families we shall use only our interview data. However, it is interesting to recall that in the survey, respondents' judgements were guided quite significantly by their assessment of whether a case was 'deserving' or not (see Chapter 1). It may well be that imputed reputation feeds into people's judgements about who counts as deserving.

When we speak about reputations in this context, we are making three important claims. First, that there is a *shared* image of each individual within a kin group. Second, that this shared image is *stable over time*. Third, we are suggesting that these shared images *matter*, in the sense that they affect how people behave towards each other. In this section we explore how far our evidence supports this view of reputation, and how such reputations affect interactions between kin. We begin first by asking: do we have evidence for the existence of reputations, in the sense that there are common images of individuals shared between different kin groups members? By definition, it is impossible to answer this question on the basis of an interview with one person alone. So at this point we are going to draw our examples from kin groups where we have more than one view. This gets us further than single interviews but there is still a limitation. Because of the way in which we selected kin for interview (see Appendix A) we cannot determine *how far* a shared image might extend within the network of available kin. Having selected our initial contact within each family, we then concentrated upon interviewing those people whom she or he regarded as close kin.

We begin with the example of Mary Jackson, whose situation we considered briefly in our discussion of generosity. The example given there – of gifts of money and goods to keep her son's household while he was out of work – was characteristic of Mary, as she was portrayed to us by members of her family. The following comment is from McNeil, one of her sons:

> *McNeil*   I thank the Lord for my mum and dad every day. The amount of times that my mum and dad's helped me out, you know. Especially to have someone like my mum to lean on. I don't know how I'd feel – I mean obviously at some time in the future she's going to die. And I don't know how I'll take it.

McNeil articulates his mother's reputation in a striking way, but the image is one which was present in our interviews with all the other members of the Jackson family. Mary herself also had a clear sense of her *own* reputation. She saw herself as a person who would always turn out to help a relative in practical ways, and who was prepared to give assistance to her closest kin under any circumstances, whatever the personal cost. This was something more than rather vaguely 'hoping' that she was seen as a person like that. Mary was able to cite the comments of other people which confirmed this as a commonly held image of herself. She reported that one of her cousins had once said to her, when she had stepped in in a crisis, 'Oh Mary, you're always there when you're needed.' A comment like this not only confirms that this image of Mary was shared widely in the family. It also indicates that it was important to Mary herself to have confirmation of it.

Reputations can, of course, be less complimentary than was Mary Jackson's. Another of our kin groups provides us with evidence of a shared image of one member which was less positive, although not seriously damaging. In the Arkright family (see Appendix A for details) the view was widely shared that Oskar was bad at managing money, with a hint that he tended to be rather profligate. As he was a young, single man in his twenties, living in his parents' home at the time we interviewed him, both his parents and his adult siblings seemed inclined to see this as a flaw, but not a serious one for the moment. This view of Oskar was presented to us, in very similar terms, by several interviewees in this family, including Oskar himself. His mother described him thus:

> *Barbara*   He's not very good at coping with his monies and, er we had on a couple of occasions just to see him through some bad patches [pause]. He's like that. He's just made like that.

Oskar's father said of him, 'He's always borrowing. He's the world's worst.' His youngest sister described how she seldom borrowed money from her siblings because she did not have any to lend in return – but that Oskar had even had to come and borrow from her on a couple of occasions. All three of them laughed when they talked about Oskar's lack of financial acumen: it clearly had achieved the status of a 'family joke'.

Though we can cite evidence like this which supports our argument that reputations do get constructed within kin groups, we also have evidence that images of each individual are not consistent in every case. In an interview situation, we can have two people conveying images of another relative which seem, at least on the surface, to be at variance. Further, we also have evidence that, in some situations, reputations are directly contested in families. The Simpson case study (see Chapter 3) provides examples of reputations being contested, in the different images of Stan's siblings portrayed by Stan, his wife and his children on the one hand, and his mother Doreen on the other.

However, the clearest example in our data set of the process of contesting reputations comes from a different kin group. Because of the sensitivity of the material here we are using substitute pseudonyms to preserve anonymity. The case concerns the reputation of a man whom we are calling Ken Wilson, as seen especially through the eyes of his sister, Joyce Miller. Joyce's own image of her brother was very uncomplimentary. This stemmed crucially from an incident around the time of their father's death several years previously, when Joyce felt that Ken had given their mother inadequate support. She particularly held it against him that he had not been prepared, as she saw it, to stay with their mother while their father was dying. She told the story like this:

Joyce When my father was actually dying, the morning he was dying, he [Ken] took my mother up to the hospital, left her there, went home, phoned me. I went up to the hospital which was right. My father died of cancer by the way. It wasn't a very nice death because it was lung cancer. And I can understand him not wanting to be there when my father actually died. That I can understand in people. But when I tried to phone him he'd actually gone out. I got no answer. So I took my mother home and I went back to his house and the neighbours told me he'd gone shopping. And it wasn't local shopping either. He'd gone miles away and it upset me. I couldn't understand him not wanting to be at the hospital. To go 50 miles shopping, you know, it's not on.
Interviewer You felt that he should have been giving you more support?
Joyce Well my mother needed him. Because she is closer to him than she is to me. But he wasn't there [pause]. She needed our kid but he wasn't there. And he was out a number of hours. And I've never forgiven him. I don't find that I *can* forgive him. [Emphasis in original.]

As a result Joyce describes herself 'not friends' with her brother any more, though she kept up appearances of friendly contact especially when her mother was present.

Joyce acknowledges that she is talking here about specific difficulties in her relationship with her brother – at that level it is an example of conflict between two individuals rather than of the construction of reputations. However, it is an issue which did go beyond the two of them. Joyce presents herself as angry 'on behalf of' her mother, who had received less support from Ken than she deserved. The implication is that the poor image of Ken is shared at least by her mother Betty, and probably also more widely. Our evidence about whether this image actually *was* shared is somewhat ambiguous. Betty Wilson actually gave us no hint of that in her interview, despite some careful if gentle probing. It is quite possible that she did indeed hold an uncomplimentary view of him, but was not prepared to reveal that in an interview. Like Jane Jones in our example at the beginning of this chapter, it may be that she felt it would reflect badly on herself as a mother to acknowledge that her son had behaved inappropriately at a crucial time in the life of this family. We simply cannot be sure on the basis of the data which we have. What we feel more certain about is that Ken himself was not aware of having a negative reputation within his family. He gave no sign at all that he was conscious of this image of himself, nor even that his sister specifically was holding something against him. Thus the evidence for the existence of a shared reputation is much weaker in this case than it is for Mary Jackson.

On the other hand, the case of Ken Wilson does underline the importance of reputations in a rather different way. In our interview with Joyce's daughter Kate, we learned about the process through which Ken's reputation was being challenged and modified. When she was asked to identify whom she would count as 'immediate family' Kate initially left out her mother's brother and then added:

> *Kate* I've got an uncle, the nearest uncle, closest is my uncle Ken, my mum's brother and his wife. Now my mum doesn't get on with them [pause]. I suppose in some ways you can be brainwashed by what your mother says [pause]. I'm sure it's six of them and half a dozen of my mother as well – I know what my mum's like.

As is clear from this extract, Kate's view of her uncle is coloured by the reputation which her mother has tried actively to establish for him within the family. It is the first thing which Kate mentions when she talks about him. Although she is sceptical about where the blame lies for the rift between her mother and her uncle, this still shapes both her image of him and her actions towards him. She says that she is happy to 'give him the benefit of the doubt' but that actually she never goes to see him, adding, 'I'd feel I was going behind my mother's back. Don't want any more aggro [laughs].'

What Kate's account shows above all else is that the image of Ken Wilson among his kin *matters*. It matters to Joyce that other people's view of him should be modified as a result of his actions. It is not sufficient that her own image is changed. His reputation also matters in the sense that it affects the way in which other family members relate to him. What we seem to have in this example is a case which demonstrates that reputations of individuals can be contested in families. When we talk about shared images, we are therefore not implying that there is always a clear consensus which is easily arrived at. But the pressure does seem to be for individuals to try to produce a common view and a shared image within that group of people which they see functioning as 'their family'.

We move on now to look at the other key element in the concept of reputation – the idea that images are stable over time. By this we do not mean to imply that they are fixed in early life and never get changed. The example of Joyce Miller and Ken Wilson shows family members in the process of modifying their shared image of one member. But we would argue that the process of change is relatively slow and builds upon the reputation which went before. Reputations are not transitory – depending for example on the last contact with that person – but are stable over quite long periods of time.

The key example which we shall use here comes from our interview with Thomas MacIntyre, a single man in his early twenties at the time of the interview. Though we do not have interviews with other members of his family, we are using this example because Thomas is unusually clear in his account of family reputation and its effects over time. However, we do have to be aware that, in this particular case, we have only one view.

Thomas talked with feeling and at length about his relationship with his father's extensive kin group, who all lived in Glasgow and whom he visited about once a year. His relationship with them was coloured by his perception that his own father was regarded as the 'black sheep' of this family – a classic expression for a particular type of negative reputation. This reputation dated, so far as Thomas could discern, from over thirty years previously when his father had left Glasgow and moved to England.

Thomas   He's seen as the maverick, he's seen as the black sheep wanting, wanting to leave Scotland in the first place. That's in 1953, 1954. He's the only one of my – he's got like seven sisters – they all stayed in Scotland, he was the only one who left. And I'm sure he's not been forgiven for wanting to leave this haven. He went down to London initially.

Though we cannot confirm that Thomas's aunts did hold this view of his father, since we did not interview them, Thomas certainly treated it as well established and indicated that it was well understood among his own immediate kin – his father and his sisters. Further, it affected his own relationship with them since he felt pressured to demonstrate an adherence to the Roman Catholic faith, which his father had explicitly rejected when he left Scotland. He described the pressure thus:

> *Thomas*   I'm a fallen Catholic, so when I go there it's questions as to, you know 'What have you been doing with your spiritual life young Thomas?' You know, 'Have you been going to Mass?' I mean, talk about peer group pressure.

In this case, not only had his father's reputation persisted over thirty years, but it had discernible effects on relationships in the next generation. We have other examples of a similar nature, in which both negative and positive reputations had remained stable over long periods of time. Mary Jackson, whom we discussed earlier, would certainly be one example of the latter.

On the basis of this evidence we would argue that individuals do acquire reputations in families and that these reputations are constructed in moral terms. What our data set does not allow us to say, of course, is how *commonly* such reputations occur within kin groups, since we were not attempting to study a representative sample of families at the qualitative stage of our research. In principle it is possible to envisage kin groups where images are not shared. There may be families, for example, in which interactions take place between different 'pairs' in a way which is relatively isolated from other kin, or where widely differing images persist over long periods of time. In such families, the concept of 'reputation' would not make much sense. On the basis of our data, we must hold open the possibility that some families are indeed like that. However, we have little indication of it among the families whom we did study, especially among our eleven 'kin groups' where our data give us the most rounded picture. The weight of our evidence from these groups points to shared, rather than individualised, imagery of other kin, though – as we have already shown – sometimes this can be contested. But even where there is disagreement about someone's reputation, there is an important sense in which that knowledge is still shared – people *know* what the competing images are, and they share information which serves to confirm or refute them.

Having established that 'reputations' do exist within kin groups and seem to have some importance, we move now to consider the questions: how do such reputations get constructed and maintained? what are the elements which go into this process? Our discussions of 'not expecting' and of 'generosity' have given us some indication of what is involved as did our analysis of legitimate excuses in Chapter 4. It would seem that reputations are not generated simply as 'ideas' about a person, but are grounded in specific events and interactions which are then accorded a particular significance in contributing to the construction of a person's moral identity. In the course of negotiating assistance, we have argued, reputations are also being constructed. At this point we shall explore the processes involved more directly, looking first at the ways in which reputations get constructed or modified in families. We shall then consider how such reputations get sustained over time.

Data on how reputations get constructed initially are inherently difficult to interpret, since the whole point about reputations is that they are part of a family's history and not normally inspected explicitly. The origins of a 'good' reputation are particularly difficult to pin down in a research study like this: people may simply have no idea how one relative came to be identified as 'generous to everyone', 'always ready to help' or whatever. In our data set, interviewees who themselves hold this kind of reputation tend to trace it to childhood and say that they based their own approach to family life on the observed behaviour of a parent. We have two particularly clear cases of this – Mary Jackson, to whom we referred above, and Tilly Trotter. Both of them had the reputation of being people who were hard-working and would always step in and help in a practical way, and both linked this explicitly with the fact that their mothers had occupied the same place in the family in the previous generation.

We do not really know how far these two women's understanding of the origin of their reputation is shared within their kin groups. But it is interesting to speculate on the possibility that some daughters or sons are marked out from childhood, as it were, as the bearers of a particular reputation across generations. The idea that reputations can be transmitted across generations is also suggested by the example of Thomas MacIntyre, whose relationship with his father's sisters we discussed above. There is a sense in which he was regarded as rather suspect by his aunts precisely because he was his father's son and therefore subject to his influence. Thomas was put under pressure to accept the religious values which his father had rejected, though he seemed to be able to resist this at least covertly. Thomas uses the same phrase 'fallen Catholic' to describe the image of both himself and his father held by his aunts. Interestingly he also uses the word 'fallen' to describe his aunts' view of one of his sisters, who was apparently regarded as a 'fallen woman' because she had had a baby without being married. This evidence that negative as well as positive reputations can be transmitted across generations suggests that the process at work is that children were being 'tarred with the same brush' as their parents – a phrase in common usage which expresses well what we are observing.

It is not only in childhood, however, that we should look for the elements which go into constructing an individual's reputation within their kin group. When people refer explicitly to the construction of reputations, especially negative ones, they usually refer to incidents in adult life. Sometimes, though not always, it is a single incident which is decisive. We have several examples in our data set of the 'single dramatic gesture' which both establishes and symbolises a particular reputation. The initial decision of Thomas MacIntyre's father to leave Scotland would be one. In this example the 'single dramatic gesture' which decisively constructed a reputation concerned breaking moral codes of behaviour which were perceived as established within the family. Sometimes, however, the gesture can directly involve the negotiation of assistance between kin – one party mishandles the negotiations and then carries a negative reputation with them subsequently. There is an element of this in the cases of Joyce Miller and Ken Wilson, or Jane Jones's relationship with her son (all discussed earlier in this chapter). Also, this characterises some of the examples discussed in Chapter 4 of people failing to get their excuses for not helping a relative accepted as legitimate by their kin. In all these situations the personal conduct of one individual, in circumstances where they were negotiating with relatives, subsequently had an impact on their family reputation.

These are some of the processes which feed into the construction of reputations. But it is equally important to understand the processes by which reputations get sustained and confirmed over time. At its most fundamental, this requires that members of kin groups *talk* to each other about third parties, test out their own perceptions, and develop the shared images to which we referred above. We have already used several examples which demonstrate that kin do talk to each other in this way. One interesting facet of this talk is that it enables people to identify and understand the foundations of reputations, even if they themselves did not have any direct knowledge. In this way, younger people have 'past history' in the family filled in for them – a mechanism which presumably ensures that a reputation is more effectively transmitted across generations.

This is visible in our data set in several examples where people 'explain' the reputation of an older relative, by referring to incidents in that relative's childhood which they could not possibly have witnessed. Claire Mitchell, for example, a married woman in her twenties with three small children, resented her own father's lack of domestic contribution to the parental household, and explained this by describing the circumstances of her father's childhood.

> *Claire*   Father does very little. He washes the dishes, but he leaves them to drain, you know, he doesn't wipe them up as well. He cuts the grass and does the garden. I've only seem him hoover up once. It's only because, I think, it's the way he's been brought up. He had a nanny when he was little. He had a brother and neither of them did anything. That's why really.

The way in which Claire tells this story makes no distinction between her father's role in her parents' household, which she has observed directly, and the organisation of his own childhood home, which clearly she did not observe. Indeed, in referring to her father's childhood, she uses the phrase 'I think', indicating that she personally is wholly identified with this explanation for his adult behaviour. We have several other examples of people referring to incidents before they were born in this way, indicating the importance and effectiveness of 'filling in past history' in the process of transmitting reputations in kin groups.

Though 'talk' is the most obvious way in which reputations get confirmed, sustained and modified, it is not the only one. We also have evidence that face-to-face interactions are an important part of the same process. One point which emerges strongly in our data set is that the active cooperation of other relatives is required, not only to *change* a reputation, but also to *maintain* one. This point is most striking in relation to very positive reputations. It seems that, even where someone is widely regarded as being 'always ready to help', they may still need other people to cooperate with their efforts in order for that reputation to be sustained.

This kind of process is not easily visible in families, but in one case in our data set, it is very apparent. This concerns Mary Jackson who, as we have already noted, had a reputation of being 'always there' and willing to help. Mary's reputation among her own kin in many ways seemed very secure and it had various effects upon the way in which other people related to her. Other relatives *expected* that she would be there in a crisis and relied upon her consistency in this. On the whole her children were rather proud of their mother but McNeil did express the view that sometimes she took on 'too much', perhaps hinting that he would feel obliged at some point to step in and protect his mother from the consequences of her reputation. Mary's reputation, and the way in which she acted consistently to reinforce it, also had an impact on her relationship with her daughter-in-law, Elizabeth Jackson, though not in entirely helpful ways from Elizabeth's point of view. She described her mother-in-law in these terms:

> *Elizabeth* She knits for the kids, she bakes. She daren't turn up here unless she fetches something with her, half a dozen eggs or something, so she feels she's giving us something every time.

Mary had also made it clear that she was only too happy to offer other kinds of assistance to Elizabeth, and indeed had been called out by her to help in crises. But Elizabeth also found this a mixed blessing and said that she had decided not to rely on her mother-in-law in future if she could avoid it.

> *Elizabeth* I've learned to keep my mouth shut from her. You know, just tell her the basic outline of things, because she tends to get annoyed if she

finds out something from somebody else [pause]. If she found that we were in the red at the bank of £3000, she'd go sky high that we hadn't approached her.

Interviewer Would she?

Elizabeth Mm – and said, you know, 'Can you help us?' Even though she probably couldn't. But she doesn't like to feel that she's been left out. She likes to feel that she's involved. But then again, she doesn't want to be nosey.

Here we have a case of someone having a clear and consistent reputation in a kin group, which has a significant impact on the way in which other people negotiate relationships with her. Among other things, she needs other people's cooperation to be able to keep up her reputation as someone who is always ready to help her family. Thus offers of assistance to her kin not only are *based upon* her reputation, but the way in which they are received will also *affect* her reputation. This tells us something important about how reputations of this kind are built up, consolidated and maintained: they need the active cooperation of other people, not only to convey the image, but also to *allow* the person to act in line with the reputation which they have developed. In the case of reputations which are more negative, the active cooperation of other people is needed if they are to be modified.

CONCLUSION: THE SIGNIFICANCE OF THE MORAL DIMENSION OF NEGOTIATIONS IN FAMILIES

We stated at the beginning of this chapter that we were turning the spotlight specifically on the moral dimensions of interactions between kin. While emphasising that the material and the moral are closely intertwined, we believe that we have demonstrated that the moral dimensions are invested with considerable significance. At the same time we have shown that the true significance is missed unless one views interaction between individuals within the context of the kin group as a whole. We have argued that the key to understanding this is to see that exchanges of goods and services are also processes in which people's moral identities are implicated. Reputations are being negotiated in these interactions, and represent the means whereby shared images of individuals get transmitted from one situation to another in families.

The remaining question is: why does a person's reputation within their kin group matter? Why does it matter to that person? Why does it matter to other people? In considering these questions we are very aware that there are also other relevant questions which we cannot even begin to answer. The process of constructing and transmitting reputations is not confined to families. In working life, in leisure activities, in the local community, some individuals do apparently develop clear and recognisable reputations. In the context of our own study, we have no way of knowing whether the reputation of an individual within their kin group is consistent with their reputation outside it. We also do not know whether the process of constructing reputations in other social settings parallels that which we have identified in families. These pose very interesting questions for research but we feel that we cannot comment on them at this point, as our own research has been confined to family relationships.

One very obvious reason why reputations are important within kin groups is that they provide the basis on which exchanges of assistance can be negotiated. Someone like Mary Jackson can be approached in all kinds of circumstances and asked for practical help, and there is a very good chance not only that she will respond positively but that she will be 'pleased to be asked' and even more pleased if she can offer. We have other similar examples in our data set where a person gets asked to do things because they have the reputation for doing them. The most striking of these examples comes from the Jones family where an aunt, whom unfortunately we were not able to interview, had become the 'family carer' early in her life and had looked after a series of elderly relatives, spending most of her adult life in this way. We introduced this case in Chapter 3, as an example of responsibilities being assigned through a process of non-decision-making. Various members of the Jones kin group told us about this aunt, and these accounts make it clear that relatives had felt able to approach her for assistance *because* she had developed the reputation as the family carer. This rings true at a commonsense level – you are not going to approach someone with a request of this kind unless you have some reason to suppose that they might respond positively. Conversely, if someone has developed a reputation for never being prepared to lend money, for example, then they are very unlikely to get asked.

Thus reputations provide a *structure for negotiations* about assistance within kin groups. It is a structure which means that people do not have to negotiate with their kin in a vacuum when they need help. Individual reputations offer guidelines about whom to approach and whom to leave alone. It is also evident that, as a consequence, people's reputations get confirmed and reinforced – if someone has developed a reputation for never lending money they will not be asked, and therefore there will be plenty of evidence that they never lend money. From the perspective of an indivdual, this means that the reputation which is generated at one point in time will affect the way in which other people treat them in the future.

We have emphasised the usefulness of reputations in providing a structure within which relatives can negotiate with each other about giving and receiving assistance. But it is equally important to recognise that they are treated as valuable in their own right – symbols of personal identity which are worth fostering. Sometimes one can see that a person's reputation brings them direct benefits. A young man like Oskar Arkright (whom we discussed above), who has a reputation for being hopeless with money, might well be suspected by his relatives of actively 'cultivating' this reputation which brings him direct benefits – no one ever asks him to lend money yet they all expect that Oskar will need to be bailed out from time to time.

In most cases the personal benefits of having a particular reputation are not so clear-cut, and probably cannot be expressed in material terms. Their importance seems to lie in the extent to which personal identities are bound up with one's family reputation. In Mary Jackson's case, which we have discussed in some detail, it was apparently really important to her to cultivate a reputation for always giving assistance to her relatives. We have several other examples in our data set of women who similarly seemed to invest a great deal of themselves in the idea that they were seen as having a generous nature, always willing to respond to another person's need especially in the family, and totally reliable in a crisis. There was, for example, Jane Ashton who described herself as naturally 'a giver' and Tilly Trotter who saw herself as the focal point for giving assistance in her kin group.

This particular kind of good reputation is rather obviously gendered in character. It is a reputation in which women specifically can invest their identities for two reasons. First, the idea of being 'the family carer', or the person who is always there to make a cup of tea in a crisis, entails domestic activities which are characteristically regarded as women's domain. Thus acquiring such a reputation is regarded as appropriate for women and seen in a very positive light – for a man to acquire such a reputation would not have the same social meaning and would be a more ambiguous comment upon him. Second, it implies a strong orientation to family and kin as a major life interest – an orientation which is socially sanctioned for women more than for men. Thus this particular kind of good reputation, which entails investing a good deal of time in kin relationships, is most likely to be characteristic of women. There may well also be a sense in which family reputations generally are more important to women than to men – though we do not feel that our data set allows us to make that kind of generalisation with confidence.

Our focus on family reputations raises a further question: *why* is a person's moral identity within the kin group important? Most people do seem to *mind* what their relatives think of them, even where they see kin relationships as fairly peripheral to their everyday lives. We would argue that the reason for this lies in the distinctive characteristics of kin group relationships, particularly in relation to one's family of origin. First, they are a set of social relationships which are not chosen and they cannot be exchanged for a different set. Second, they are quite literally life-long: they are established on the day you are born and will last as long as all the parties are alive. Unlike friendships, which require some active willingness on both sides to maintain them, kin relationships have an element of permanency which is independent of their quality at a personal level. Third, these very characteristics give a social 'place' to each of us which defines an element of identity in an important way, even though subsequently we develop other elements of our identities which are not tied to the family into which we were born (see Finch, 1989: 221–36). Finally there is a more instrumental reason. To the extent that family relationships do provide a set of people to whom one can turn for assistance if other sources fail, we all have an interest in keeping on good terms in case we need to draw upon such assistance in the future. Thus the instrumental and the symbolic reasons for cultivating a good reputation reinforce each other.

Thus we are each locked into a particular set of kin relationships without the prospect of changing them for a more congenial set if they prove too difficult – as we can do with friendships. We *have* to go on interacting with our kin (at least at some minimal level), especially with those who are genealogically close and very obviously 'ours'. Therefore it matters that we sustain a reputation which makes future interactions not too difficult. Of course there *is* the choice of withdrawing totally from contact with kin, and this is indeed a choice which some people exercise. But most people do not, even if they find their relatives a bit of a trial. In those circumstances contact may be kept to a minimum but, while at least this level of contact is maintained, reputations matter. And while one's reputation within the family matters, individuals are bound to be subject to a degree of constraint in their actions towards relatives. The kin group as a whole, through the shared images which its members hold and transmit, has the power to confer or withhold a 'good' reputation. Hence it is not enough for any of us to behave properly towards our relatives according to our own criteria. It is vital to have our actions *accepted* as appropriate and for that view to be translated into reputational terms. It therefore becomes understandable why, as we have emphasised throughout this chapter, the moral consequences of negotiations within families are often treated as more important than the material ones.

6 Conclusion

INTRODUCTION

A 'Conclusion' to this type of book can mean different things. Some authors provide a helpful summary and overview of the book's contents, a condensed guide to the findings of the study. We are not attempting that kind of conclusion. With a very rich data set, analysed with reference to some difficult theoretical questions, we feel that we could not summarise the complexities discussed in preceding chapters without compromising them or misrepresenting them. Instead we have chosen to make this a more substantive conclusion. We are using it to draw the key strands of our argument together, in order to make explicit the distinctive view of family responsibilities at which we have arrived, and to consider some of its implications.

We do this in as straightforward a way as possible, without referring again to our evidence or to other research. Readers who want that kind of detail will need to consult earlier chapters. Some of the ideas developed here (and elsewhere in this book) link with the discussion in Janet Finch's *Family Obligations and Social Change* (1989), a book written on the basis of existing published work and before we had analysed our own data. Other arguments developed in this book diverge from it. The distinctive task which we are setting ourselves here is to present an argument about the nature of family responsibilities which is grounded in our empirical data, though naturally it is informed by the work of other people and by ideas developed previously.

FAMILY RELATIONSHIPS AND FAMILY RESPONSIBILITIES

We began by posing questions about the nature of kin relationships and responsibilities: how significant are kin as sources of practical and financial assistance? Do people accept that they have a responsibility to provide such assistance for relatives, or at least for certain relatives? Does the concept of 'family responsibilities' have any real contemporary meaning? Should all these questions be answered differently for women and men? We are now in a position to give some answers to these questions, and we want to highlight three elements of our analysis: (a) the significance of kin relationships as social support; (b) the nature of kin responsibilities; (c) material and moral dimensions. We follow this section with some brief comments about the broader implications of our analysis.

The significance of kin relationships as social support

The empirical evidence from our qualitative study shows kin relationships to be a significant source of assistance for many people. Most people have experience of money being lent or given, even if this involves quite small amounts in most cases. Many people have experience of living in a household which was shared with an adult relative (who was not part of a core nuclear family), at some point in their lives. Many have helped to look after someone who was ill or incapacitated, or been on the receiving end of such assistance. Some have also looked after a relative's children, given practical help with the house, the garden or the car, or given emotional support to a relative who was feeling fragile. In Chapter 2 and Appendix C we have given details which indicate the range of such experiences among our study population of eighty-eight people. At the simplest level, our study updates the work of researchers who looked at family and kinship in Britain in the 1950s and 1960s (Young and Willmott, 1957; Bell, 1968; Rosser and Harris, 1968; Firth, Hubert and Forge, 1970). They concluded that, despite widespread beliefs to the contrary, the extended family was alive and well, and had a tangible reality in most people's lives. We are saying that, thirty years later, it still does.

However, our main point is not so much that these experiences of giving and receiving help within families were *common* experiences (though many of them were), but that they were treated as *unremarkable* experiences by many people who talked to us. They were seen as a characteristic part of family life. They form part of people's image of what constitutes 'a family' and most people in our study wanted to claim that they were part of 'a family' of this type. They were keen to show us that their family did actually work as a support system for its members, at least at a minimal level. We have suggested (in Chapter 2) that the minimal level is defined as everyone rallying round in a crisis to give practical and moral support. We have just one or two exceptions to this in our study population but for the most part our interviewees said that their own families worked at least at this level. Of course there were plenty of examples of conflict, or of people not actually receiving help when they felt they needed it. And our interviewees were very aware that some families appear to work better than others as support systems. But almost all of them presented their own family as 'working' at the minimal level at least, even if they also had indicated that they saw their own family as 'less close' than some others.

To put the point slightly differently, we are arguing that the kin group *is* seen as something which you can fall back on if things go wrong in your life, especially if there are unexpected traumas or disasters. But it is a safety-net which should be used as a last resort, not as a first resort. People expect that, for most of their adult lives, they will *not* be drawing on the support of kin apart from their spouses. Indeed much of our data shows people trying to *avoid* relying on help from relatives, rather than routinely expecting to call on it. Many people go to great lengths to ensure that they do not become dependent on this type of assistance (see especially Chapter 2).

So we are arguing that, while most people value a kin group which 'works' as a support system for its members, most can only be actually relied upon to do so in sudden crises and in situations of 'last resort'. In other circumstances our data suggest that the kin group is much more unreliable as a support system, at least when looked at from the outside. By this we mean that it is not possible to predict, simply from knowing the genealogical relationships, what kind of support is likely to be given to any individual. Knowing that Mr X has a brother, or five sisters, or two sons, does not enable me to say if he is likely to be looked after when he is ill, lent money if he needs to replace his car, or given a temporary home if his own household is split up by separation or divorce. Some brothers, or sisters, or sons would offer any of these forms of help; others would not. The offers of help do not flow straightforwardly from the genealogical relationship. Certainly it is more likely that parents and children will help each other – particularly down the generations, from parents to adult children – than will other relatives. That is clear from the evidence contained in Appendix C, and our survey data endorse people's beliefs that it *should* be so (see Chapter 1, and also Finch and Mason, 1990b, 1991). But even support from parents or children is actually very variable in practice.

Are these variations accounted for by other social characteristics of the individuals involved – their gender, their occupations, their ethnicity, their incomes? In previous chapters we have firmly rejected the idea that these kinds of 'structural factors' explain the help which passes in families in any straightforward way. Of course people who are in comfortable financial circumstances have more options about helping their relatives than do families where everyone is on the breadline. In that very simple sense, some of our variations are accounted for by people's economic and social circumstances. But the idea, for example, that working-class people in general are more inclined to value family support than are the middle classes

– or indeed the other way round – simply does not square with our data, either the survey data or those based on qualitative interviews. One reason why 'structural factors' do not straightforwardly explain people's experience of giving and receiving help, is that they are in part a *product* of help given and received in the past. For example, parents' assistance to their children in getting them through higher education, in helping them to set up businesses or to buy houses, or to migrate to another country, all have an effect upon the occupational class position that the children occupy in adult life. Thus factors such as occupational class or housing tenure cannot be regarded as 'independent variables' in this context.

Two exceptions to this argument are ethnicity and gender because, except in very unusual circumstances, these are fixed at birth. In this study, we wanted to explore ethnic variations but were unable to do so effectively in the survey data (see Appendix A). In our qualitative data we have eleven interviewees out of eighty-eight who were of Asian or Caribbean descent – a number large enough to give us some indication of where the similarities and differences might lie, but obviously not the basis for making detailed and generalisable comparisons. In fact we are struck more by the similarities in the experience of our white interviewees and those of Asian or Caribbean descent, than by the differences between them. Certainly we can identify some obvious differences. For example, in kin groups of Asian descent, we found evidence of a continuing expectation that a son, rather than a daughter, will take responsibility for giving a home to elderly parents – though the labour of caring for infirm elderly people will largely fall on women in the household, as in the white community. But other than this kind of difference, built on specific or cultural norms about the responsibilities of kin, the ways in which our black and Asian interviewees (all of whom were young adults who had been brought up in the UK) approached family responsibilities had many similarities with those of the white people we talked to.

In relation to gender, there certainly are some differences but not of a simple kind. At the level of publicly expressed beliefs, women and men say essentially similar things about the value which they place upon assistance between kin and the circumstances in which it should operate. Therefore any differences in women's and men's involvement with their kin cannot be explained by the idea that they hold different beliefs about the family or adhere straightforwardly to different value systems. When it comes to looking at what happens in practice, women in general do seem to be more firmly locked into sets of responsibilities to relatives, and men are more peripheral. However, here, as with all our data, we find considerable variations between individuals and exceptions in both directions.

In this section we have sketched out the basic pattern which shows that kin relationships *are* significant as structures of social support, but in a variable way. In subsequent sections we refer to these patterns and attempt to develop our understanding of them.

The nature of kin responsibilities: rules, rights and commitments

The concept of responsibilities lay at the heart of our research agenda in this study. Where we find examples of people giving assistance to their kin, does it make sense to talk in terms of responsibility or obligation or duty, associated with family relationships specifically? This question links with the theoretical debate (see Chapter 1) about whether in general kin relationships have a special character which marks them off from all others, and are distinctively defined by obligations and responsibilities. In essence, our answer is that the patterns of assistance which we have identified *are* underscored by a sense of 'family responsibility', but that we have to look carefully at what this means.

We need to clear away first of all what it does *not* mean. We found very little evidence to support the view that people see specific duties attached to family relationships. Our main purpose in the survey element of our study was to see if it is possible to identify anything approaching rules of obligation which are widely acknowledged at the level of publicly expressed norms. We found that there are not. The variations which we observed in practice, in the assistance which relatives give to each other, also suggest that responsibilities do not operate on the basis of fixed rules. The interviewees who came closest to talking about rules of obligation on the whole were people of Asian descent but even here, as we have noted, there were variations in how that worked out in practice. For most people responsibilities towards relatives were not fixed. They are far more fluid than the notion of 'rules of obligation' implies. To return to the distinction which we made in the introductory chapter, the concept of 'guidelines' seems to fit our data much better than 'rules'. Further, the guidelines which people recognise are procedural rather than substantive – they indicate how to work out whether it is appropriate to offer assistance to a particular relative, rather than ones which point to what you should do in concrete terms. It is for these reasons that we have chosen to use the word 'responsibilities', which perhaps has less of a sense of fixed rules than does 'obligations' or 'duties'.

So we would argue that the idea of 'duty' is an inappropriate way of thinking about family life. We would reject even more strongly its corollary, 'rights'. If there were fixed rules of obligation or duty in families, then we might expect that one person felt a duty to give assistance and the other felt a right to claim it. But our data show a particularly strong resistance to the idea that anyone has a right to claim assistance from a relative (see especially Chapter 5). This is one of the strongest messages in our data and is supported, in different ways, by evidence from the survey and from the qualitative study. Claiming rights is definitely not seen as a legitimate part of family life. Even where one person accepts a responsibility to help, the other does not have the right to claim, or even to expect, assistance. We have argued that this is because the right to offer help must always remain with the donor – particularly important in a situation where there are no fixed rules of obligation. The fact that responsibilities are not mirrored by rights reinforces our basic point that they are fluid and not fixed.

So in what sense *can* we identify responsibilities within kin groups? Our most important point here is that a sense of responsibility for helping someone else *develops* over time, through interaction between the individuals involved. It is a two- (or more) way process of negotiation in which people are giving and receiving, balancing out one kind of assistance against another, maintaining an appropriate independence from each other as well as mutual interdependence (see Chapters 2 and 3). As a product of these processes, one individual becomes committed to giving assistance to another. Responsibilities thus are *created*, rather than flowing automatically from specific relationships.

We have referred to the process of creating responsibilities as one of negotiation between individuals. Sometimes the negotiation is explicit but often it is not. The outcome of such negotiations is not fixed in advance, but at the same time it does not take place in a vacuum. Though there are no fixed rules about *what* should be given to relatives there are some well understood guidelines about *how* such negotiations should be conducted. We saw this reflected in our survey data, in the fact that we found more procedural than substantive consensus (see Chapter 1). Our qualitative data also show, for example, that there are some well understood principles which can be used by people in prioritising the various claims upon their time, their money or their labour (see Chapter 4); also principles concerned with how to conduct oneself in negotiations, above all the importance of not *showing* that you expect help (Chapter 5).

We have found the concept of *developing commitments* particularly valuable in expressing the processes which we are uncovering. It is a conceptual framework which both helps us to understand the processes involved in negotiating responsibilities, and also helps to explain why we find the kind of variations which our data display. We are using the concept of commitments as developed originally by Howard Becker (1960) and we explain this in some detail in Chapter 3. The essence of this idea is that people develop commitments *over time* and in ways which are possibly half-recognised but often not consciously planned. One person helps another out in a crisis and the other then wants to return the favour. Opportunities for doing this may occur easily or they may not. Where a pattern of reciprocal assistance builds up over time, each person invests something of themselves in *this* relationship and becomes committed to it as a relationship through which mutual aid flows. The essence of becoming committed, in Becker's terms, is that it becomes 'too expensive' to withdraw from the situation which is developing. The 'expense' is not necessarily calculated in material terms, though it can be. This was certainly the case in one or two instances in our data set where, for example, someone got locked into a set of commitments to an older generation because they were to inherit property and money when that person died. But more usually, it seems, the expense is calculated in terms of people's personal identities and their moral standing in their kin group and in the eyes of the world at large.

Thus the concept of developing commitments encapsulates much of what we have said about the ways in which family responsibilities are created between specific individuals over a period of time. It also helps us to understand why we have such a pattern of variation in people's experiences of assistance in kin groups, and in the pattern of responsibilities which they acknowledge. Such variations occur because responsibilities are a product of interactions between individuals over time. The course which such inter-actions take can be very variable even for members of the same family, including people in the same genealogical position (as sons, sisters, grandmothers or whatever). At the same time, the genealogical relationship of individuals does play some part in shaping the course which such interactions are likely to take. For example, we have argued that parent–child relationships – particularly 'down' the generations – come closest to being in a category of their own. However, we see the explanation for this as located within the framework of 'developing commitments', rather than the idea that fixed rules of obligation cover parent–child relationships. What we are saying is that the conditions under which people live their lives make it more likely that parents and children will develop commitments to each other, but that the underlying processes of developing commitments are the same for all categories of kin.

To understand why parent–child commitments appear strongest 'down' the generations, we think that we need to take account of the social relations of child-rearing which prevail in this society. Parents are allocated responsibility for young children in a sense which is public as well as private, sometimes directly a matter of public policy. When children are young, parent–child relationships are *defined as relationships* in which parents take responsibility for the material and emotional welfare of their children. We are suggesting that the effects of this may flow into adult life, making parent–child relationships down the generations the only relationships in which someone can be held morally 'accountable' for how someone else 'turns out' in adult life. In a sense then, the conditions conducive to developing commitments are set from childhood. This will be the case much more commonly for parents and children than for other kin. But the point is that the processes would be the same for all categories of relative, even though the conditions under which people live their lives make it much less likely that cousins will develop stronger commitments than, for example, parents and children, or siblings. As we have shown though, sometimes they do, and even within the parent–child range, there is great variation in the responsibilities which people acknowledge.

We think that we can understand the role of the structural location of individuals in the way commitments develop in similar fashion. For example women, who conventionally are seen as having time more readily available than men, are more likely to get locked into sets of commitments which entail giving time and labour. So responsibilities, as we have said, do not get negotiated in a vacuum but they do get negotiated in ways which allow for considerable individual variation. At the same time we would argue that such variation should not just be seen as idiosyncratic and incomprehensible. The concept of commitments helps us to put a framework on it and to understand how such variations come about.

In defining family responsibilities this way, as created and not predetermined, we recognise that we could be describing processes through which a person develops a sense of responsibility to *anyone*, not just to members of their family. So are we saying that there is nothing distinctive about *family* responsibilities – that they are just one example of a more general process through which one human being becomes committed to helping another? Ultimately we cannot answer these very interesting questions about the difference between responsibilities towards friends and responsibilities towards relatives because we have not done a comparative study of the two. But looking solely at our data on family relationships, the fact that people are related genealogically does seem to create distinctive elements in the process of developing commitments to kin.

Chief among these is the sense that a person 'belongs' to their kin group in a way which is not true of other social groups of which they might be a member. Especially in relation to the family of origin, a kin group is the group into which a person is born, in which the membership is in no sense chosen, and where relationships still exist throughout life even if they are left dormant. It therefore exists as a ready-made context within which responsibilities can appropriately develop, and also are very likely to develop as people interact with each other. It is precisely the same set of features which also makes the kin group an appropriate safety-net to use as a last resort. In *this* sense kin relationships *are* distinctive.

Material and moral dimensions of family responsibilities

One distinctive feature of the argument which we are developing is to emphasise the interweaving of what we are calling the material and the moral dimensions of family life. Though this is perhaps implicit in earlier research, in analysing our own data we have come to see the importance of bringing this into the foreground.

Essentially our argument is that it is not possible to understand the nature of family responsibilities, or how they operate in practice, if you concentrate only on their material dimensions and look at exchanges of goods and services solely in terms of their material value. Certainly such exchanges *are* 'reckoned' in material terms, but only up to a point. In order to see their full significance, and to understand the dynamic which such exchanges create and recreate, we have to also see the moral dimensions. By 'moral dimensions' we do not mean moral rules. We have already indicated that the evidence of our study leads us to reject the idea of following moral rules, as an inappropriate way of describing how family responsibilities operate. When we talk about seeing the moral dimensions of family responsibilities, we mean that people's identities as moral beings are bound up in these exchanges of support, and the processes through which they get negotiated.

Much more is at stake therefore, than simply the material value of the goods and services which are exchanged. People's identities are being constructed, confirmed and reconstructed – identities as a reliable son, a generous mother, a caring sister or whatever it might be. The concept of commitments links in here too. If the image of 'a caring sister' is valued as part of someone's personal identity then it eventually becomes too expensive to withdraw from those commitments through which that identity is expressed and confirmed. It appears that a particularly important aspect of identities constructed in relation to family responsibilities is the dependence–independence dimension. It has been a strong theme in our data (see especially Chapter 2) that most people strive to ensure that they do not beome 'too dependent' upon assistance from relatives. A certain degree of interdependence is allowed, indeed is highly valued. But any situation where one person receives more than they can return to the other is definitely to be avoided.

Thus our argument is that, through negotiations about giving and receiving assistance, people are being constructed and reconstructed as moral beings. In thinking about the ways in which people's identities form part of these interactions, we have found it useful to talk about 'reputations'. In Chapters 4 and 5 in particular we have developed the idea that people's reputations are at stake in all instances where a need is responded to or not responded to. A person's identity or reputation gets confirmed or modified as a result of the way in which they conduct themselves on each occasion. Reputations, we have argued, are not simply the image which one individual has of another, but they have a more public and a more enduring character. Reputations are images of each individual which are *shared* by members of their kin group (and possibly by other people too) and they have an influence upon the course of future relationships. By stressing that reputations are shared rather than individual images we do not mean to imply that there is always total agreement. In Chapter 5 we have shown that there are cases where a person's reputation within their family is a matter of some dispute. But in a sense this reinforces our point that a person's reputation is public not private property. It is moulded and remoulded as that person's actions are observed and talked about by other members of their kin group.

In focusing on these moral dimensions of family life we also see very clearly the potential for conflict and for outcomes which do not suit one or more of the parties. This is an important counterbalance to our evidence that, on the whole, people do want to see themselves as part of a family that 'works' at least at a minimal level, and make some effort to ensure that it does. But when we see how closely people's identities and reputations are bound in with kin exchanges, it seems very unlikely that families are going to 'work' equally for all people all of the time. The ways in which they 'don't work' can vary. We have noted that there certainly are some examples of people in our study who have received little from their kin and have given little (see Chapter 2 and Appendix C). Family responsibilities seem to have a marginal place in the lives of these people and the family may not 'work' as a support system, even of last resort.

There are also ways in which the family 'doesn't work' for individuals on a moral level, even when it does seem to be working at the level of material assistance. The clearest of these examples arise when an ongoing process of exchanges between kin leaves one person 'beholden to' another. This can happen in a whole range of circumstances – where a young person has to rely on their parents' financial assistance after they feel they should be fully independent; in old age when a person may become physically dependent; at the end of a marriage when an adult child returns to the parental home, in need of moral support and assistance with child care. In such circumstances, it is possible in principle for the person in the position of donor to extract forms of repayment which might otherwise not have been given. 'Moral blackmail' is a phrase commonly used to describe such situations, and indeed it was used by some of our interviewees. In earlier chapters we have quoted a few examples which do seem to amount to a fairly naked exercise of such power. More commonly people do not actually take advantage of these situations in this way – indeed they may be careful to avoid opportunities to exercise the power which potentially they have. But this does not really change the situation fundamentally for the person who has become the net recipient in an unbalanced pattern of exchanges. Their identity and their position within the kin group has changed, and they *are* beholden to someone else, even if this is not openly acknowledged. The strenuous efforts which people make to try to avoid getting into such situations demonstrates how unwelcome this is.

We have emphasised the importance of the moral dimensions in understanding how family responsibilities operate but we do not mean to imply that the material dimensions are of no importance. In terms of the practical consequences of kin group exchanges, they are exceedingly important. The quality and standard of living of individuals can be enhanced or eroded in very significant ways through exchanges between kin of money, goods, labour and time. Also the material value of assistance is taken into account in 'reckoning' the moral dimensions of exchanges. We see this very clearly when we look at how people try to keep a balance between dependence and independence in relationships with their kin. Some very fine calculations (which of course may not be successful) take place to try to ensure that no one becomes a net giver or net receiver, or is beholden to someone else. The way such calculations are reckoned centrally concerns the material value of the exchanges.

In summary, our purpose is not to argue that the moral dimensions of exchanges are more important than the material, or vice versa. Our central theme is that the two are finely interwoven. To see either without the other is to miss the main point.

SOME BROADER IMPLICATIONS OF OUR ARGUMENT

Our main purpose in this chapter, as we have indicated, is to provide a clear statement of our argument about family responsibilities, based on the empirical study which we have undertaken. Having done that, we are very aware that our arguments have more general implications. We happen to have studied kin relationships but the processes which we have uncovered may well have parallels in other social settings. At this level we connect with some rather important issues in sociological theory. We shall indicate briefly what we think these are. It would be inappropriate to make any serious attempt to develop these here – to treat them properly would require extended discussion. Therefore we are not referring to or elaborating upon the relevant sociological literature in this section. Our aim is simply to identify these broader issues and to point up some of the questions which, we believe, our work raises.

The central sociological issue to which our work connects is the debate about social structure and human agency, and how the two relate. These debates essentially are concerned with the question: how can we understand the processes through which people create and make sense of their own lives, yet do so within constraints which they have little or no power to alter? In treating 'responsibilities' as created commitments rather than rules of obligation, we are saying firmly that they are the product of human agency and not an external property of social structure over which individuals have no control. But there is also a sense in which they become structural features, in that they both constrain and facilitate future actions. On the one hand they make it possible for one person to draw upon the assistance of another, in ways which they could not do without the development of reciprocal commitments. On the other hand they place limits on the range of options subsequently available. Thus we think that our study provides an empirical example of the *processes* through which agency and structure relate.

While placing our emphasis on agency we believe that we have also said that social structure *is* important. But we think that we are using a concept of structure that is more fluid than that often found in sociological writing. We can illustrate this by considering the idea that each person has a 'structural position' which shapes the kind of commitments which they can negotiate with others, and influences the likely outcome of such negotiations. Conventionally in relation to kinship, each individual's structural position would be defined by genealogy and by gender: a mother, a father, a brother, a sister and so on. Such definitions 'place' individuals in relation to other relevant individuals.

In our view this is not enough if you want to know what is one person's effective structural position in relation to other kin, at any given point in time. We refer here to 'effective' structural positions to emphasise that we need to know, not only formal definitions, but also what those positions actually mean – *how* they are going to constrain human agency. We would argue, on the basis of our data, that we need to look also at *what each person has accumulated* over time. We certainly need to do this in a material sense. If one daughter has accumulated property and wealth but another has not, this puts them in different structural positions *vis-à-vis* their elderly parents. Such concerns conventionally are linked with social structure. But we believe that we also need to look at what someone has accumulated morally – their identity, their reputation, their commitments. Certainly in the context of kinship we need a concept of 'structural position' which incorporates these facets, if we wish to understand how human actions are constrained at any given point in a person's lifetime.

If we are right, then it is possible that this more fluid concept of social structure is more widely applicable. How far does what someone has accumulated – morally as well as materially – define their effective structural position in other social settings? Occupational settings are one obvious example, especially those in which 'professional reputations' seem to play an important part. Political and voluntary activities are another. Can accumulated commitments to support your local Conservative Club, or the group trying to prevent the building of a nuclear power station, be analysed in the same way as commitments to relatives? Is a reputation as 'a good Labour party member' or 'a faithful Catholic' something which both shapes and constrains action in the ways which family reputations do?

This brings us to our final point about the structure versus agency question. This concerns the processes through which people construct and use social meanings – one aspect of human agency in operation. In planning our research project we looked at this issue slightly differently. We made a clear distinction between beliefs and actions and argued that in order to understand family responsibilities, we need to look at both. In the design of our project we felt it important to ensure that we did not make the error of 'reading off' people's likely actions from the beliefs which they express about family relationships, particularly in answer to survey questions. We still think that was absolutely right. To make a simple link of that kind would be a fundamental mistake.

However, in analysing our data, and developing the argument which we have presented, we found that we were using the dichotomy of 'beliefs versus actions' less and less. This is because we have increasingly realised the importance of looking at the ways in which social meanings are constructed *for use* rather than seeing them as ideas which exist inside people's heads. Beliefs, in that sense, may or may not exist. Increasingly we have come to the conclusion that it is a mistake to concentrate on the question: 'what does this person "really believe"?' If what we are trying to do is to understand how social life actually operates, that question probably misses the point. What matters is to understand the meanings which his or her actions *convey* to other people. We have reached this conclusion through several strands in the analysis of our empirical data. In Chapter 4 we saw the importance, in relation to particular events and needs within families, of each person's developing a position which others would regard as legitimate. Our examples in that chapter focused upon what we called 'legitimate excuses', on situations where a person was trying to avoid giving assistance to a relative – lending money, offering them a home, looking after their children or whatever it might be. Whether or not someone could *successfully* establish a legitimate excuse could be the crucial factor in determining whether they did end up giving assistance or not. The question of whether someone 'really believes' that they have a responsibility to help this particular relative is not very relevant here in understanding why they do or do not give assistance. Much more important is how their actions are going to be understood by other people. In Chapter 5 we showed that, more generally, having your actions understood 'in a good light' is important in the process of developing responsibilities and commitments.

It is through these kinds of data that we have come to appreciate that the meanings which social actions *convey* may be a much more important topic for study than attempting to understand what the authors of those actions 'intended'. This is not an original idea but, if it is more generally applicable, it has some interesting implications not least about research methods. As it happens our own research design made it relatively easy for us to pick up the importance of this feature of social actions because we collected data from a number of different individuals in the same kin group. Project designs which make this kind of perspective possible seem essential for any researcher who wishes to understand the social meanings actually conveyed by actions.

These are the main points which we want to make about the connections of our work to larger sociological questions. We are finishing this section by commenting briefly on the implications of all this for the analysis of gender relations. In a sense gender offers one example of how the more abstract theoretical arguments, which we have developed above, would apply to a substantive aspect of social life. But gender cannot be treated as just one example among many. As is well recognised in all the relevant literature, gender divisions and gender relations are absolutely fundamental to the patterns of family responsibilities which most people develop in practice. To make no comment on it would be to leave a very important end untied.

So, what are the implications of our analysis for understanding gender relations? We think we have demonstrated that the processes of developing commitments and responsibilities to kin *are* gendered but not in the simple kind of way that is often supposed. In general women are more firmly locked into sets of family responsibilities than are men, and usually more finely tuned to issues of negotiations, identity, reputation and the like. But there is considerable variation for both women and men. We feel that we cannot say that in practice someone accepts a responsibility 'because' she is a woman – or even because she is a daughter – when there is so much variation and when people themselves do not present their actions in that way. We relate our argument at this point to what we said above about the concept of 'structural position'. Being 'a daughter' is only part of what constitutes someone's effective structural position. We also have to know – for each individual – what she has accumulated in the course of her life, both materially and morally. One daughter may have accumulated a far more extensive range of commitments than others, even her own sisters, and these form part of the structural position which a woman occupies at any point in her life.

Similarly we think it too simple to argue – as some feminist literature does – that women and men adhere to different sets of moral values, and that this explains why they handle responsibilities differently. As we said in our general comments on the concept of 'beliefs', we do not find it very useful to think about people 'holding' sets of beliefs or values in a rather static way. Rather we think that we should focus on the meanings which women and men successfully *convey* to others with whom they negotiate. Thus the important question is not: do women and men really believe different things about family responsibilities? It is: are there differences in the way people perceive and interpret the actions of women and men towards members of their family? Do women have more difficulty than men in getting certain positions accepted as legitimate?

In essence we are arguing that the differences which we observe between the patterns of responsibilities acknowleged by men and those acknowledged by women do not result from holding different sets of ideas, or even from occupying different structural positions, as conventionally understood. We would argue that these differences *emerge* as women and men negotiate their own relationships with their relatives. Over a period of time, the differences get established and – since commitments established at one point affect future negotiations – they tend to get consolidated.

The processes of developing commitments, which we have uncovered, enable us to understand how commitments do get consolidated once a person has begun on that path. But there remains the question: why is it usually women rather than men who *begin* on a path which leads to more extensive sets of responsibilities? Though we cannot explore these issues in any depth here, we would argue that the explanation lies in the very different conditions under which women and men live their lives more generally. On the whole women are more likely than men to *need* to develop sets of reciprocal commitments with relatives because they are still more likely to be allocated the major responsibility for the care of children and the management of a home – matters where it is quite difficult to get help from other sources and where help from relatives is considered appropriate. Equally, women are less likely to have the sort of consistent record of employment in well-paid jobs which gives the basis of a life-time's financial independence. Because women are more likely to be in a position – and perhaps anticipate that they are going to be in the position – where they need the kind of assistance which kin can provide, they are more likely than men to begin on a path in early adult life where they start to develop sets of reciprocal responsibilities with kin. But it is certainly possible – as one or two instances in our data set show – that a man can be in analagous circumstances. Where, for example, a young man has received significant economic assistance from his kin to enable him to set up a business, this could be the kind of situation conducive to a man's developing sets of commitments to kin on a scale more commonly associated with women (though of course they may be commitments of a different *type*).

This very sketchy outline of the kind of ideas about gender relations implied by our analysis obviously has broader implications which cannot be considered here. Our main point is to highlight the importance of understanding accumulated commitments in women's lives particularly, and of seeing this as a feature which significantly shapes the actions which they take. We would argue that theories of gender relations need to be capable of accommodating the variations in experience which flow from this kind of process. They need to give due weight to human agency, rather than seeing the experience of women and men as flowing directly from the different structural positions (as conventionally defined) which they occupy.

IMPLICATIONS FOR SOCIAL POLICY

It has not been our purpose in this book to examine policy issues and policy options directly. However, as we noted in our introduction, the work which we have been doing raises questions about the ways in which the concept of family responsibilities gets incorporated into social policy. We are going to finish by identifying these questions. We are not going to elaborate on the background to the relevant policy issues, as we have discussed this in some detail elsewhere, especially in Finch (1989). However, we feel that we can comment now with some authority because we can base our analysis on a recent and extensive data set.

The questions which we want to address centre round a comparison between contemporary social policies – in particular the assumptions that are made about the nature of family responsibilities – and the way in which people think about and act towards their relatives in practice. As we indicated in Chapter 1, governments have to draw the line somewhere between the responsibilities of the state for supporting its citizens, and those needs which it assumes will be met by the family. If families are meeting their members' financial and practical needs, then there is no necessity for governments to get involved. If they are not, then it may be necessary to make provision through state funds and facilities. In planning these, governments need to make some assumptions about what most families will provide and what they will not. It can be shown that, in periods when governments are trying to keep down the cost of public expenditure, there is an incentive to encourage families to provide as much as possible (Crowther, 1982). One such period, it can be argued, was the 1980s when the British and many other Western governments tried to re-draw the boundary between state responsibilities and family responsibilities to place more in the realm of the family. Increasingly kin were seen as the first line of assistance for most people with the state playing a residual role (see Finch, 1989, for an elaboration of this argument).

However, the place at which that line is drawn has to be realistic, in the sense that it needs to take some account of the expectations which most people do really have, concerning what it is reasonable for family members to provide. Our data enable us to compare the points at which that line currently is being drawn with the ways in which family responsibilities operate in practice.

Our first point of comparison concerns the concept of family responsibilities itself. Social policies in Britain have long operated with a view of responsibilities which sees them as a 'natural' property of relationships between spouses, between parents and children, and possibly beyond that. The Victorian Poor Law expressed this most directly, in the way in which it allocated financial responsibilities for maintaining named categories of relatives – spouse, immature child or grandchild, elderly parent. People could be required through law to acknowledge these responsibilities in practice. Built on an earlier tradition, it was not seen as an attempt actually to change the way in which families operate. It was based on the assumption that it was 'natural' for relatives to acknowledge these responsibilities towards each other and that their codification in law simply expressed something which all decent people would be doing in any case. Such codification makes it possible for governments to *assume* that certain services will be provided by the family, and therefore to draw a clear line at the point where the responsibility of the state begins. However, it also implies a role for the state in enforcing family responsibilities where individuals are reluctant to accept them, which did indeed occur under the Victorian Poor Law though not always with total success (Crowther, 1982; Quadagno, 1982). Thus there is a history within British social policy of governments acting in a rather contradictory way when drawing the line between family responsibilities and state responsibilities. On the one hand it is assumed that certain forms of reliance upon relatives is a 'natural' part of family life. On the other hand it is accepted as part of the state's role to enforce such responsibilities – which implies that they are not universally regarded as natural.

Our data suggest that any notion that specified responsibilities are 'natural properties' of named relationships is well out of step with the contemporary reality of family responsibilities and the way they are arrived at. Quite possibly this has always been so – a conclusion which would be consistent with the fact that governments in the past found it necessary to devise ways of enforcing responsibilities which it presumed to be natural. One of the most important messages from our data is that the responsibilities which people acknowledge are variable and do not flow straightforwardly from particular geneaolgical relationships. There is no guarantee that 'a son' or 'a sister' will feel responsibilities of a specific kind. We have argued that responsibilities between kin grow out of, and are dependent upon, the history of particular relationships. It makes little sense therefore to build public policies which assume that certain types of assistance will be given more or less automatically. Support may well be offered – but its availability will vary from one family to another and from one individual to another. This is a normal feature of family life, not a sign that some people are irresponsible or uncaring.

Perhaps even more important than our argument about variability is another strong message from our data: people do not want to have to rely on their relatives for extensive help. We have found clear evidence of active avoidance of, sometimes resistance to, accepting help from a relative. It has been a long-running theme in the study of elderly people's family relationships that they seek 'intimacy at a distance' – a relationship with their children and grandchildren which is close at an affective level, but where they do not have to rely on them too much on a daily basis and maintain a strong sense of their own independence (Townsend, 1965; Wenger, 1984; Finch, 1989; Qureshi and Walker, 1989). Our data not only offer further confirmation of this but also show that it is not simply elderly people who want to maintain independence from their relatives, and strive hard not to rely on them too much – it applies to young adults, to people in middle age, to both men and women, every bit as much as it does in the case of elderly people. All try to ensure that they do not get into situations where they are 'beholden to' relatives.

What we have found, in effect, is a continuing and strong sense of individualism in social life which, it can be argued, has long characterised English society. As Macfarlane's (1978) influential work on this topic makes clear, Britain has had a distinctive social and economic structure at least since the thirteenth century, of which individualism is a key component. It has been accompanied by a model of family life in which kin relations outside the nuclear family were relatively unimportant, by comparison with other societies in western Europe. In England, the expectation that people will keep themselves economically and practically separate from their kin has roots which go back at least six centuries. This evidence directly challenges any idea that the family should be seen as the first and most appropriate line of support wherever possible, and that the state should simply play a residual role, perhaps concentrating assistance mainly on people unfortunate enough not to have relatives. Policies which are designed to make people *more* dependent on their relatives breach a principle which many people hold dear.

Our final point about social policy concerns the idea that people should have the right to fall back on assistance from their relatives. The idea of 'rights' to assistance was expressed explicitly in the Poor Law concept of 'liable relatives'. These were people identified as having a duty to offer assistance to a relative in need, and the corollary of that duty was the the right to make claims upon such assistance. In England a person had the right to make claims for financial assistance upon a spouse, a son, an unmarried daughter or (if they were a child of immature years) a parent or grandparent. In Scotland this was extended further to a grandchild, a brother or a sister (Wall, 1977; Crowther, 1982; Quadagno, 1982). The concept of liable relatives was removed from the law in 1948, leaving legal liability only between spouses, and for young children. However, the more that governments try to re-draw the boundaries between the state and the family, and to extend the range of responsibilities which they assume will be taken by kin, the closer we come to reviving the idea of liable relatives (whether or not the same term is used).

The idea that anyone has the 'right to claim' help from a relative is well out of line with our evidence about how family life operates. People reject even the idea that anyone has the right to *expect* assistance, let alone to *demand* it. The right to provide or withhold help must always remain with the potential donor, we have argued. This is a principle to which people adhere strongly, both in theory and in practice. There is a strong resistance to any suggestion that a potential recipient ever has the right to make claims.

The clarity of our data on this point should act as a strong indication that policies which rest on the assumption that people have a right to expect assistance from their relatives (even from their parents or their children) will not align with the realities of family life. People *do* accept responsibilities to help relatives, sometimes at considerable cost to themselves. But we all, it would seem, want to retain the right ultimately to say that we do it of our own choosing. Our study has shown that 'family responsibilities' operate in a way which is much more complex and more individual than the idea that we acknowledge and follow rules of obligation. It simply doesn't work like that.

Appendix A: Methodology and research design

The Family Obligations Project was funded by ESRC, grant number G00232197: £121,000, 1985–1989. The study used a two-stage research design, involving a large-scale survey, and a smaller in-depth qualitative study. The rationale for this research design is described in Chapter 1.

THE SURVEY

The survey was designed by Janet Finch in consultation with Social and Community Planning Research (SCPR). It involved structured interviews with 978 respondents. SCPR undertook the data collection and preparation, between September 1985 and February 1986.

Full details of the sampling procedure and technical aspects of the survey are given in Gill Courtenay's *Survey of Family Obligations: Technical Report*, London, SCPR, February 1986. This is available from the authors for consultation on request.

Sampling

The survey was carried out in the Greater Manchester area among a representative random sample of adults aged 18 and over. The response rate among those who were eligible for interview was 72 per cent (978 respondents). Sampling was executed using a two-stage, stratified, cluster sampling technique. Forty-five electoral wards in the Greater Manchester region were selected from a list ordered according to the OPCS Constituency File, and using a random start number and a fixed interval. Within each selected ward, thirty-five addresses were selected with equal probability from the 1985 Electoral Registers. This procedure yielded a sample of 1,400 addresses. In order to convert the sample of addresses to one of individuals, the names of all electors were listed for each address, and the name of the individual on whom the sampling interval landed was marked with an asterisk (this person is known as the 'starred elector'). The interviewers then called at the address of each 'starred elector' where they listed all those eligible for inclusion in the sample (that is, all people aged 18 and over). When the list of eligible people and the list of electors for the address were identical, the interviewer attempted to interview the 'starred elector'. But when the list of eligible people differed in any way from the electors registered for that address a random selection was made using a Kish Grid.

Sample characteristics

The following tables set out our sample characteristics by comparison with appropriate national data, and data from the Greater Manchester District. Our purpose in making these comparisons is to allow readers to develop a view of the representativeness of our achieved sample. We believe that we have achieved a sample which is reasonably representative of the national population, with small variations on a few of the characteristics. However, the sample is not necessarily representative of sub-groups of the national population which appear in small numbers, such as respondents from non-white ethnic groups.

Table A.1 Gender

| | Sample | | Greater Manchester 1981 | National Data 1981 |
	Frequency	%	%	%
Male	429	44	49	48
Female	546	56	51	52
Missing	3			
Totals	978	100	100	100

Source of national data: OPCS, 1982, 1983. All figures based on adult population aged 18 and over.

Table A.2 Age

	Sample		Greater Manchester * 1981	National Data 1981
	Frequency	%	%	%
18–29	223	23	27	23
30–49	342	35	32	34
50–64	224	23	22	23
65 and over	184	19	19	20
Missing	5			
Totals	978	100	100	100

Source of national data: OPCS, 1982, 1983.
* Greater Manchester figures here are based on the age range 16 upwards, so are not directly comparable with sample and national statistics which are based on 18 upwards.

Table A.3 Ethnic group

	Sample*		National Data** 1983–5 Combined
	Frequency	%	%
White	955	98	95
Asian	5	0.5	2
West Indian/African	9	1	1
Other	1	0.5	2
Missing	8		
Totals	978	100.0	100

Source of national data: OPCS, 1987. National data are based on a sample of adult population aged 16 and over. Sample is based on adult population aged 18 and over.
* Based on interviewer's assessment of ethnic group.
** Based on interviewee's assessment of ethnic group.

Table A.4 Economic activity: percentage economically active or inactive

	Sample	National Data 1985
Men		
Economically active	74	67
Economically inactive	26	33
Totals	100	100
Women		
Economically active	48	54
Economically inactive	52	46
Totals	100	100

Source of national data: OPCS, 1987. All figures based on adult population aged 18 and over.

Survey questionnaire content

The survey questionnaire used the vignette technique (see Finch, 1987a) to ask questions about three main types of support between relatives: personal care, accommodation and financial support. This involved posing hypothetical situations concerning third parties, and inviting respondents to indicate what should be done in those situations. Most of the questions had both precoded and open coded parts. Appendix B gives examples of the short vignettes used in the survey. The questionnaire also included four longer vignettes, in which respondents were guided through an evolving hypothetical situation, and asked what should be done at specified stages. The following is an example of one of these vignettes.

> John Highfield is a married man in his early thirties. He and his wife have two young children. John is unemployed but has a chance to start his own business. He can get various grants to help him get started, and the bank will lend most of the money he needs. But he still needs another £1,500.
> (a) If he thought his parents could afford to help, should he ask them for the money?
>> Yes.
>> No.
>> Don't know/depends.
>
> *If answer is yes:*
> (b) Should he ask them for a gift or a loan?
>> Gift.
>> Loan.
>
> (c) Why do you think he should ask for a gift rather than a loan (or loan rather than a gift) ?
> *Probe fully and record verbatim*
>
> *Ask all*
> (d) He does not like to ask his parents for the money, but should they offer it?
>> Yes.
>> No.
>> Don't know/depends.

(e) John's parents do offer the money. But John knows that his father's pension is low and that the money will come out of his parents' small savings account. Should John accept the money or should he refuse it?
>> Accept.
>> Refuse.
>> Don't know/depends.

If accept or refuse
(f) Why should John accept/refuse the money?
Probe fully and record verbatim

The logic and rationale of using vignettes in the survey is outlined in Chapter 1. Basically, the intention was to tap public norms or statements about 'the proper thing to do' in specified circumstances. We did also include some general questions about family responsibilities and obligations. We did not intend to use the survey to discover what people actually did in practice, and therefore we only asked a few limited questions about respondents' own experience of giving or receiving the three types of support. These were contained in a more general section about respondents' social characteristics, which was used to construct variables for analysis.

THE QUALITATIVE STUDY

The qualitative study also took place, for the most part, in Greater Manchester. A few interviews were conducted elsewhere in the north west region of England. These involved respondents of Asian or Caribbean descent whom we contacted via a different sampling strategy. A few others took place in other parts of England, because we were interviewing relatives of respondents living in Greater Manchester. Both of these aspects of our sampling strategy are explained more fully below.

This part of the research was designed and conducted by Janet Finch and Jennifer Mason, and data collection took place between 1986 and 1988. The qualitative study involved 120 interviews with eighty-eight people; thirty-one of these had also taken part in our survey, and most of these respondents were interviewed twice at the qualitative stage. Our policy was to interview our initial contact person in any family twice, if they agreed. Mostly, these were the people who had also been in the survey (see sampling strategy below) but seven had not. These seven were respondents of Asian or Caribbean descent, who were included in the qualitative study via a different sampling strategy (see below). The remaining interviewees were interviewed only once, usually because they were included in the study as kin of our initial interviewees (see below).

Policy on confidentiality

All interviewees are referred to by pseudonyms throughout this book. Interviewees were invited to choose their own pseudonyms, and most of them did so. Some people selected names which are those of fictional characters or of people in real life: we have not altered these. Furthermore, in some of our discussion, we have felt it necessary to use additional measures to preserve anonymity. We have done this in a number of ways: by changing pseudonyms; by changing characteristics or events in a way which does not alter the analysis; by using examples abstracted from their context and/or without a pseudonym attached at all.

Sampling

Our sampling strategy was guided by the principles of theoretical sampling, and we have discussed this fully in Finch and Mason (1990a). We did not aim to produce a sample representative of the general population in statistical terms. Instead we wanted to end up with a study group which would help us to understand the processes of negotiation about responsibilities between relatives. This meant incorporating into the study group people who might have been involved at some stage in processes of negotiation and renegotiation of family relationships. We wanted to capture a range of experiences, or instances of negotiation and support, and we sampled accordingly. Initially, we decided to use our survey as a sampling frame. Respondents in the survey had been asked whether they would be willing to be contacted again, and we used those who said yes as our starting point. We began by selecting people who were either young adults, or who had been divorced or separated, on the basis that these two groups would have experience of the negotiation and possibly renegotiation of family relationships. We were not seeking straightforwardly to compare the experience of young adults and divorced people, but were using both groups as a 'way in' to the kinds of family situations which we did want to study.

We subsequently engaged in two 'stock-taking' exercises (several months apart), designed to examine our study group and its characteristics and experiences, and to modify our sampling strategy on that basis. The major principle which we used to guide our selection at those points was theoretical signficance: we chose to focus on those groups and experiences which would enable us best to evaluate and develop the theoretical ideas and concepts with which we began the project. The approach we adopted was intended to achieve that, by being both flexible and systematic. Details of the study group are given below.

Another important strand in our sampling strategy was the inclusion of relatives of our initial interviewees. Where an interviewee was married, or cohabiting, we asked whether we could approach their partner for interview. If they agreed, we usually did a second interview with the initial respondent, and a simultaneous interview with the spouse in a different room in their own home. Forty of our interviewees have a spouse or cohabiting partner in the study.

Additionally, with some interviewees, we asked if we could approach other relatives. We made these requests at the end of the second interview with the initial interviewee. We have called our successful examples of this 'kin groups'. We have eleven of these in our study group, where we interviewed between three and eight members of the same family. In all, fifty-eight of our interviewees have kin other than a spouse in the study. We felt this was important, given our focus on processes of negotiation between relatives: including a number of members of the same family would help us to understand negotiating processes from different perspectives and positions. We followed up the kin of our initial interviewees using similar criteria of theoretical significance, but also we made our selections within the range of kin that our initial interviewee had identified as close, or important, or immediate kin. Therefore, kin groups 'belong' to the initial interviewee (see Chapter 1, and Finch and Mason, 1990a, for elaboration of these points). The 'shape' of our kin groups as a result depends first upon who was named as close or immediate kin, and second upon whom out of that list we wished to interview and agreed to be interviewed.

It is important to add that we made a policy decision not to attempt to gain access to people whom we knew to be in 'crisis' situations, on ethical grounds. Details of the kin groups are given below.

Another aspect of our sampling strategy concerns the mechanism by which we included people of Asian and Caribbean descent in the study group. Our method of using people who had taken part in the survey as initial interviewees in the qualitative study failed to give us access to any people of Asian or Caribbean descent, for a combination of reasons. As stated above, these groupings formed only small proportions of our survey respondents and that factor, added to a higher refusal and non-response rate, meant that none of them ended up in the qualitative study. This was because: either they did not fit our theoretical sampling criteria (we did not want to pick any respondent fitting the description of Asian or Caribbean descent, if they did not display any of the other characteristics or experiences in which we were interested); or they declined to be interviewed; or they were no longer living at the same address and we could not trace them.

So, we had to adopt a different strategy, and this involved using personal contacts to get introductions to people of Asian or Caribbean descent. This strategy took us away from the Greater Manchester region, and these interviews were conducted in other parts of north west England. In total, we did twelve interviews with seven people; two of Caribbean descent, and five of Asian descent. All of these were young adults. We were similarly unsuccessful in gaining access to either an Asian or Caribbean kin group, although we do have interviews with two brothers of Asian descent (Mohammed and Rafiq Hussein).

Qualitative interview content

The qualitative study involved semi-structured interviews which were tape recorded and fully transcribed. Interviews lasted on average around one and a half hours. We were interested in people's own experiences of family relation-ships and responsibilities, and the negotiation of support within families. Hence we asked people about such experiences, inviting them to couch their responses within a life-history framework. Although we followed up similar themes in each interview, in a sense each interview comprised its own parti-cular focus, namely the specific experiences, relationships and responsibilities of that interviewee. As a result, we did not ask exactly the same questions of each interviewee, and the interview products are not directly comparable on those terms (see Appendix C where this point is elaborated).

Study group characteristics

We set out below various key characteristics of our study group, and show the gender distribution for each of these. In addition, we have identified into which categories our respondents of Asian and Caribbean descent fall. Our main purpose in setting out these characteristics is to give a sense of the *range* of people we interviewed at the qualitative stage. We are not making claims about the representativeness or otherwise of the study group on the basis of these characteristics.

Table A.5 Gender

	No. of Respondents	%
Female	49	56
Male	39	44
Totals	88	100

Interviewees of Asian descent: 2 female, 3 male.
Interviewees of Caribbean descent: 1 female, 1 male.

Table A.6 Age

	Men	*Women*	*Total*	%
18–29	14	16	30	34
30–49	14	18	32	36
50–69	7	12	19	22
70+	4	3	7	8
	39	49	88	100

Interviewees of Asian descent: 4 aged 18–29, 1 aged 30–49.
Interviewees of Caribbean descent: 2 aged 18–29.

Table A.7 Current paid employment status

	Men	Women	Total	%
Full-time employed or self-employed	28*	15	43	49
Part-time employed or self-employed	–	10	10	11
Retired	6	6	12	14
Unemployed or other not economically active	4	13	17	19
Student	1	5	6	7
Totals	39	49	88	100

* Includes one Asian man on YTS scheme, and one white man on Enterprise Allowance scheme.
Interviewees of Asian descent: 3 full-time, 1 part-time, 1 student.
Interviewees of Caribbean descent: 1 full-time, 1 student.

Table A.8 Current occupational group (for those currently in employment)

	Men	Women	Total	%
Professional	4	3	7	13
Employers and managers	5	2	7	13
Other non-manual	6	13	19	35
Skilled and semi-skilled manual	9	5	14	26
unskilled manual	5	2	7	13
Totals	29	25	54	100

Interviewees of Asian descent: 2 other non-manual, 1 skilled or semi-skilled manual, 1 unskilled manual.
Interviewees of Caribbean descent: 1 skilled or semi-skilled manual.

Table A.9 Educational qualifications: highest qualification

	Men	Women	Total	%
Degree or equivalent	9	5	14	16
Higher education	3	5	8	9
'A' levels/equivalent	3	3	6	7
'O' levels/equivalent	7	12	19	22
CSE/equiv/commercial or apprenticeship	4	8	12	13
Other qualifications	1	1	2	2
No qualifications	12	15	27	31
Totals	39	49	88	100

Interviewees of Asian descent: 1 with 'A' levels, 1 with 'O' levels, 3 with CSE/equivalent.
Interviewees of Caribbean descent: 1 with 'A' levels, 1 with 'O' levels/equivalent.

Table A.10 Housing tenure: people living in households which are:

	Men	Women	Total	%
Owned with mortgage	20	23	43	49
Owned outright	11	14	25	28
Privately rented	5	5	10	11
Local Authority rented	1	6	7	8
Other	2	1	3	3
Totals	39	49	88	100

Interviewees of Asian descent: 3 owned with mortgage, 1 owned outright, 1 privately rented accommodation.
Interviewees of Caribbean descent: 2 in privately rented accommodation.

Table A.11 Religion

	Men	Women	Total	%
Christian	22	36	58	66
Hindu		1	1	1
Moslem	3	1	4	5
None/not specified	14	11	25	28
Totals	39	49	88	100

Interviewees of Asian descent: 1 Hindu, 4 Moslem.
Interviewees of Caribbean descent: 2 Christian.

Table A.12 Political allegiance

	Men	Women	Total	%
Conservative	9	10	19	22
Labour	13	14	27	31
Lib/SDP	4	13	17	19
None/not specified	13	12	25	28
Totals	39	49	88	100

Interviewees of Asian descent: 2 Labour, 3 none/not specified.
Interviewees of Caribbean descent: 1 Labour, 1 none/not specified.

Kin group details

We have eleven kin groups in our study, involving interviews with between three and eight people in any one kin group. The following gives brief details of each of the kin groups and its members. In line with our policy on confidentiality, all names are pseudonyms, and most were chosen by the interviewees themselves. Usually the initial interviewee chose a family name and other interviewees simply chose a first name. Where there is more than one family name within a kin group, subsequent family pseudonyms were usually chosen by the first interviewee with a different family name from our key interviewee.

The Yates: Sarah Yates's kin group

We interviewed six members of this family, beginning with *Sarah Yates*, a 42-year-old married woman who lived with her second husband and their 15-year-old daughter, in their own home in the Greater Manchester region. Sarah was employed full-time as a driver. Her second husband, *John Yates*, was our second interviewee. He was aged 59 and had worked as a mechanical engineer for over thirty-five years until his 'early' retirement in 1986. Since that time he has done part-time voluntary work. He and Sarah had been married for sixteen years at the time of our interviews with them. Our next interviewee was Sarah's daughter by her first marriage, *Anna Yates*. Anna was aged 22, and lived with her boyfriend in another part of north west England. She had left her parental home to train as a nurse.

We also interviewed Sarah's mother, *Ethel Phillips*, a 73-year-old widowed woman who lived near to Sarah and John, and also near to Sarah's brother. Ethel did factory work before she had her children, and various part-time jobs afterwards including working as a cleaner and in a canteen. She retired from her last job in 1986. Sarah's brother, *Henry Phillips*, was our fifth intervieweee in this kin group. A married man aged 49, he and his wife live about three miles away from Sarah's household. He is a self-employed decorator, and he and his wife have two teenaged children.

Finally, we interviewed one of Sarah's cousins, whom she had identified as a close relative. *Mary Mycock*, aged 37, lives with her second husband, her two children aged 10 and 8 from her first marriage, and one of her husband's children, aged 21, from his first marriage. Her husband's other child, a daughter aged 19, used to live with them also but has now left home. Before the birth of her children, Mary did full-time clerical work. She does not intend to return to full-time employment until her children are at secondary school. Mary's household is also in the Greater Manchester region.

The Archers: Shula Archer's kin group

We interviewed five members of this family, beginning with *Shula Archer*, a 19-year-old single student living in her parents' home. Shula had been doing an 'A' level course, but in between her first and second interviews with us she left the course, and went to work and live in a Kibbutz in Israel for a short period. Shula had a brother aged 13, and two sisters aged 6 and 4, none of whom were included in our study. We did interview Shula's parents, *Jill Archer* and *Phil Archer*. Jill and Phil were married, and neither had been married before. Both were 'only' children. Jill was aged 43, and employed from time to time as a supply teacher, although she saw herself as most fully engaged in bringing up her children. Phil was aged 42, and self-employed full-time as a partner in a practice of veterinary surgeons. They lived in their own house in Manchester.

We also interviewed two of Shula's grandparents, *Dorothy O'Malley* and *John O'Malley*. Aged in their late sixties and early seventies respectively, these were Jill's parents, and they lived in the Manchester region also, although in a different town from Jill, Phil and Shula. Both had retired after a life-time's working in a public service industry. We did not interview Shula's other grandparents, that is Phil's parents, who lived also in Greater Manchester, and were aged 80 and 79.

The Simpsons: Julie Simpson's kin group

We interviewed four members of this family, beginning with *Julie Simpson*, a 25-year-old single woman who lived alone in her own flat in Manchester, where she had moved after completing her degree course at a university in the Midlands. Julie was employed full-time as a computer programmer. Her parents, *Stan Simpson* and *Eileen Simpson*, also took part in our study. They lived in Leeds in their own house, which they shared with Stan's widowed mother, Doreen, who did not take part in our study. Doreen had been living in the household for eighteen years. Stan and Eileen were aged 52 and 46 respectively, and they had recently acquired a grocery shop which they were running together. This followed Stan's redundancy from a management post a few years previously. Eileen had not worked full-time for many years prior to taking on the grocery shop, but had done a number of part-time jobs including shop work.

Julie had two younger sisters, one of whom – Clare – had been married and divorced, and was now living with her new partner in Essex. Clare remained in Essex when her parents and sisters moved from there to Leeds, following a promotion for Stan. She married shortly afterwards. Clare did not take part in our study. Julie's other sister, *Janet Simpson*, was our fourth interviewee in this family. She was aged 21, single, and lived alone in a privately rented flat in the same town as her parents. She had moved out of her parents' household about a year before our interview with her. She was employed full-time as an insurance clerk locally.

The Kings: Avril King's kin group

We interviewed just three members of this family. *Avril King* was our initial contact. She was married, aged 43, and lived with her second husband and their 13-year-old son in their own home in Greater Manchester. Avril and her husband had been married for twenty-three years (she married for the first time about thirty years ago). She was employed part-time doing shop work. Avril's husband, *Miles King*, was our second interviewee. He was aged 52, and was employed full-time in a public service industry. Miles had not been married before.

Our final King interviewee was Miles's father, *Alfred King*, a 77-year-old twice-widowed man. Alfred had remarried after the death of Miles's mother, and had two adult stepchildren from his second marriage, as well as another son from his first. He lived in his own home not far away from Miles and Avril. He was now retired, but had been a railway worker throughout his working life.

The Crabtrees: Jean Crabtree's kin group

We interviewed six members of this kin group, beginning with *Jean Crabtree*, a 24-year-old single woman who lived with her partner in a house which they jointly owned in the Greater Manchester region. Jean was employed full-time doing clerical and secretarial work. Her partner, *David Waterworth*, was our second interviewee in this kin group. David was 23 years old, and was employed full-time as a computer representative and consultant. Jean and David planned to marry in a year or two's time.

Jean had a brother and a sister. Her brother was aged 37 and lived in the north west of England, but did not take part in our study. Jean's sister, *Joyce Stevens*, also lived in the Greater Manchester region, and did take part. Joyce was aged 39, married with two children aged 13 and 8, and was not currently in paid employment. Jean and Joyce's widowed mother, *Ellen Crabtree*, was also one of our interviewees. Ellen was aged 63, and lived alone in a flat she had purchased under a sheltered housing scheme, in the north west of England. Ellen's husband, Jean's father, had died some twenty years before, following which Ellen retrained as a book-keeper and gained full-time employment. All of Jean's grandparents had died, but she had three remaining uncles; one, her mother – Ellen's – brother, and the other two her father's brothers.

Jean also identified some of her quasi in-laws as close kin, and David's mother and father, *Tom Waterworth* and *Ethel Waterworth*, also took part in our study as a result. Aged in their late forties, they lived in a small town in a different part of north west England, where they ran a fish and chip shop, which also provided their rented accommodation. One of David's sisters (single and aged 18), and his brother (single and also in his late teens), lived in the parental household, and David's third sister (single and aged 21) lived nearby with her 2-year-old child. Tom and Ethel had run a series of small businesses over their life-times, including an hotel in a British seaside resort, and a bar in Spain. They lived in Spain for a few years, along with all their children with the exception of David, who remained in the UK. All of David's grandparents had died, but he had two uncles; his mother's brothers.

The Arkrights: Simone Arkright's kin group

We interviewed seven members of this kin group, beginning with *Simone Arkright*, a 22-year-old single woman who lived in her parents' household in Manchester. Simone was employed full-time in an insurance company. She had five siblings: two sisters and three brothers. We interviewed all but her eldest sister (who was in fact the eldest sibling) who was aged 26, married and living in Canada where she worked as a shop manager. The youngest sibling whom we interviewed was 20-year-old *Selina Arkright*, Simone's other sister. Selina also lived in the parental home, and was at college doing a business studies course at the time of our interview with her. She was single, but had just become engaged. *Dylan Arkright* and *Eric Arkright* were twins aged 23. Dylan lived in the parental household, and was employed full-time as a graphic artist. Eric had moved out of the family household after doing a degree course at university, and now worked for the Ministry of Defence in the south of England. *Oskar Arkright* was the eldest brother. He lived in the parental household and worked as a lab technician in a local hospital, but planned to leave home shortly to seek work abroad.

Our other two interviewees from this kin group were Simone's parents, *Barbara Arkright* and *Kenneth Arkright*. They were married, and had not been married previously. Barbara was 60 years old, and worked as a night sister in a special baby care unit in a local hospital. Barbara was born and brought up in Ireland, where three of her sisters (one brother had died, and the other sister lived in London) and their widowed mother still lived. Kenneth's origins were in Manchester. He was 75 years old, and had retired from his job as a warehouse manager some fifteen years prior to our interview with him. He had not taken paid work since that time. Both of his parents were dead, as were four of his six siblings.

The Mansfields: Susan Mansfield's kin group

We interviewed six members of this kin group, beginning with *Susan Mansfield*, a married woman in her mid-thirties with four children aged 20, 17, 13 and 7. The eldest two, a son and a daughter, lived away from home and were from her first marriage. The younger two lived at home, and were from Susan's second marriage. Susan lived in Manchester with her second husband in their own home, and she worked as a data preparation officer. Her husband, *Roger Mansfield*, was our second interviewee. Roger was aged 36, and was a full-time student at a local university. He had not been married previously. One of Susan's brothers, *Kevin Ellis*, was married to one of Roger's sisters, *Kath Ellis*. We interviewed both Kevin and Kath. They had four young children, and lived in their own home just round the corner from Susan and Roger. Kath was not currently in paid employment, and Kevin had been made redundant from his job in the steel industry. Roger had four other siblings, one of whom, *Lesley Trafford*, we interviewed. She was aged 40, married with two children aged 20 and 16, and ran her own 'corner shop' business in the Greater Manchester area. Susan had one other sibling, a brother, whom we did not interview.

Roger's father had died in 1985, but his mother, *Nan Mansfield*, was aged 67, living locally in her own home, and also participated in our study. She did not have paid employment. She had separated from her husband – Roger's father – some years before his death. Her own mother had died when she was very young, and she had been brought up by an aunt, who had also died some years ago.

The Jacksons: Robert Jackson's kin group

We interviewed five members of this kin group. *Robert Jackson* was our first interviewee. He was aged 37, and living with his second wife and their two young children in a rented house in the Greater Manchester region. Robert had recently taken 'early retirement' from a public service occupation on grounds of ill-health, and was in the process of setting up his own business. He had a daughter aged 11 from his first marriage with whom he had little contact. David's second wife, *Elizabeth*, was our next interviewee. She was aged 27, and did not have paid employment although she had done various part-time jobs recently – including shop work, pub work and catering. Elizabeth had not been married before, and she and Robert had been married for five years.

We then interviewed Robert's parents, *Richard Jackson* and *Mary Jackson*. Richard was aged 68, and Mary was aged 67. Neither had been married before and they lived together in their own house in a different part of Greater Manchester from Robert and Elizabeth. Richard had worked for the local authority for many years in manual occupations, until his retirement in 1979. Mary had worked part-time as a seamstress and retired in 1983.

McNeil Jackson, one of Robert's two brothers, was our final interviewee. He was aged 40, married, and lived in a different town in north west England with his second wife and their two children aged 9 and 7, and his son aged 18 from his first marriage. McNeil had recently started his own business in home improvements, having left a public service occupation.

The Frosts: Andrew Frost's kin group

We interviewed six members of this kin group, beginning with *Andrew Frost*, a 23-year-old married man. Andrew lived in Manchester with his wife, in their own house. He was employed full-time as an accountant, and became fully qualified shortly after our second interview with him. Andrew's wife, *Elizabeth Frost*, also took part in our study. She was aged 24 and was employed full-time as a secretary. She and Andrew met while they were at Manchester University, both doing degree courses. Andrew was born in the Midlands. He left his parental home in order to go to university, and did not return again afterwards. Elizabeth was born in South Wales, and similarly left home to attend university and did not return afterwards. Elizabeth's father died in 1979, but her mother still lives in South Wales, as does her brother and her sister, both of whom are married.

Andrew's parents, *June Frost* and *Francis Frost*, both took part in our study. They are married, neither having been married previously, and live in the Midlands in their own house. June does not have paid work, but Francis is employed full-time as a physicist. Francis's mother is alive and lives locally, but his father, and June's parents, have all died.

Andrew also has two siblings, both of whom were interviewed as part of our study. *Jack Frost* is his elder brother. He was in his early thirties when we interviewed him, married with a baby, and living in London in a house he and his wife owned jointly with another couple. Jack was employed as a company secretary, full-time, and his wife worked part-time as a trading standards officer. *Jane Smith* is Andrew's elder sister. Also in her thirties, she is married with two young children. Jane trained as a teacher, but is currently not in paid employment, and neither is her husband. They live in their own home in the Midlands, in a different town from Jane's parents.

The Gardners: Tim Gardner's kin group

We interviewed three members of this family, beginning with *Tim Gardner*, a 22-year-old single man who lived in privately rented accommodation in Manchester which he shared with friends. Tim had until recently been a full-time university student, and following on from that a sabbatical officer for the Students Union. After that, he started a small business selling second-hand and handmade clothing on a market stall. Tim was an only child. His mother, *Caroline Gardner*, who also took part in our study had been involved in Tim's business venture as a dressmaker and adviser. She and her husband, *Lawrence Gardner*, our third interviewee in this family, lived in Greater Manchester in their own home. They were aged 50 and 51 respectively when we interviewed them. Caroline from time to time did part-time paid work, mainly dressmaking, for a variety of employers. Lawrence was a self-employed upholsterer, in a family business he had inherited from his father. His mother had died in 1982, and his father in 1987, shortly before our interview with Lawrence. Caroline's parents had both died, her mother fairly recently, and her father in 1968. Lawrence had one married sister, who lived locally, and Caroline was an only child.

The Joneses: Isobel Jones's kin group

We interviewed five members of this, our final, kin group. The first was *Isobel Jones*, a 42-year-old widowed woman. She lived in her own home with her son. Her daughter had recently left home. Isobel had a full-time professional job in the education sector. She had been widowed for about two years. Prior to that, she and her husband and their two children had lived in South America for about six years in the 1970s. Isobel had a married sister who lived in Canada, and who did not take part in our study.

Isobel's son *Zaki Jones* was our next interviewee. He was aged 22, and was a student. He was living at home temporarily in between a degree course and a Master's course, both at universities away from north west England. He had also done various part-time and temporary jobs. Zaki's younger sister, *Ann Jones*, was our next interviewee. She was aged 20, and had recently moved out of her mother's household to share a local authority rented flat with friends nearby. She had worked on a YTS scheme, and had recently started 'A' level courses.

We also interviewed Isobel's mother, *Kathleen Snow*, a 62-year-old widowed woman who lived nearby in her own home. She had not been in paid employment for many years. Kathleen had just one sister who lived nearby but who did not take part in our study. Isobel also identified her late husband's mother as close family, and we interviewed her also. *Jane Jones*, herself a widow, was in her seventies, and lived nearby in another part of Greater Manchester. She lived in a house which had been provided by her late husband's employer, and where she had been allowed to remain since his death in 1976. Jane also had not had paid employment for many years.

Appendix B: Should relatives be the preferred source of help for someone in need of assistance? Survey findings

Appendix B gives details of the survey findings discussed in Chapter 1. These relate to fourteen questions from the Family Obligations Survey, where we sketched out a situation where a person was in need of assistance, then asked respondents to say whether the help should come from relatives or from some other source. We have selected only shorter questions for this exercise. The survey also contains several longer and more complex questions, where choices of this type are posed. Data from the longer vignette questions are discussed elsewhere in the book.

In this appendix we are giving the question wording, followed by the frequencies. We have also noted the consensus baseline (explained in Chapter 1) for each question. Details of how the survey was conducted can be found in Appendix A and in Chapter 1.

We have grouped the questions in the following way:

A. Questions where there was a high level of agreement that help *should* come from relatives.
B. Questions where there was a high level of agreement that help *should not* come from relatives.
C. Questions where there was a split pattern of responses.

A. HIGH LEVEL OF AGREEMENT THAT HELP SHOULD COME FROM RELATIVES

1. Suppose that a couple with a young child have returned from working abroad and can't afford to buy or rent anywhere to live until one of them gets a job. Should any of their relatives offer to have the family in their own home for the next few months?

	Frequency	*% of respondents*
Yes	842	86.1
No	80	8.2
Don't know/depends	56	5.7
Total	978	100.0

Consensus baseline: 75%

2a. A 19-year-old girl, who has been living with her boyfriend, has a baby. She and her boyfriend split up and she can no longer go on living in his home. She cannot afford to rent a home of her own. Should she:

	Frequency	*% of respondents*
Go back to her parents' home	774	79.1
Do something else	133	13.6
Don't know/depends	67	6.9
NA	4	0.4
Total	978	100.0

Consensus baseline: 75%

2b. (Respondents who said 'something else' or 'depends'.)
Do you think that her parents ought to offer her a home or not?

	Frequency	*% of respondents*
Yes	154	77.0
No	42	21.0
Don't know/NA	4	2.0
Total	200	100.0

Consensus baseline: 75%

B. HIGH LEVEL OF AGREEMENT THAT HELP SHOULD NOT COME FROM RELATIVES

3. A young couple with children aged 2 and 4 have not been able to have a holiday since the children were born. They want a two-week holiday but cannot afford it. Should they:

	Frequency	*% of respondents*
Try to borrow from the bank or some other organisation	170	17.4
Try to borrow the money from relatives	150	15.3
Do without the holiday	654	66.9
Don't know/NA	4	0.4
Total	978	100.0

Consensus baseline: 50%

4. A young couple with children aged 10 and 8 want to send them to a private school but cannot afford the fees themselves. Should they:

	Frequency	*% of respondents*
Try to borrow from a bank or other organisation	166	17.0
Try to borrow the money from relatives	30	3.1
Keep the children in state schools	772	78.9
Don't know/NA	10	1.0
Total	978	100.0

Consensus baseline: 50%

C. SPLIT PATTERN OF RESPONSES

5. If someone has enough money to help an elderly relative who cannot look after himself or herself, which of these three forms of help do you think would be best?

	Frequency	*% of respondents*
Pay for the relative to go into a nursing home	161	16.5
Pay for someone to help in the relative's home	452	46.2
Help the relative themselves	288	29.4
Don't know/NA	77	7.9
Total	978	100.0

Consensus baseline: 50%

6. Are there any circumstances under which it is reasonable to refuse to provide personal help for a sick or elderly relative?

	Frequency	*% of respondents*
Yes	564	57.7
No	363	37.1
Don't know/not sure	51	5.2
Total	978	100.0

Consensus baseline: 75%

7a. Suppose a young couple need an extra £800 for the deposit on their first home, and they cannot borrow the money from a bank, building society or loan company. Should they wait to buy a home until they have got enough money, or should they see if they can borrow it from relatives?

	Frequency	*% of respondents*
Wait until they have enough money	606	62.0
Borrow from relatives	341	34.9
Don't know/depends	31	3.1
Total	978	100.0

Consensus baseline: 75%

7b. (Respondents who said 'wait' or 'depends'.)
Are there any circumstances under which you think it would be alright to borrow from relatives?

	Frequency	*% of respondents*
Yes	322	50.5
No	313	49.2
NA	2	0.3
Total	637	100.0

Consensus baseline: 75%

8. If someone lends money to a relative so that they can start a business, do you think that the loan should be repaid with interest, or should just the amount that was borrowed be returned?

	Frequency	*% of respondents*
Repaid with interest	404	41.4
No interest	503	51.4
Don't know/depends	71	7.2
Total	978	100.0

Consensus baseline: 75%

9. If a student runs up £400 in debts while at college, do you think that parents should pay off the debts, even if it means some financial hardship for them?

	Frequency	*% of respondents*
Parents should pay	239	24.4
Parents should not pay	638	65.2
Don't know/depends	101	10.4
Total	978	100.0

Consensus baseline: 75%

10a. If an elderly person wants to go into a private nursing home to live, but can only afford part of the price, do you think that relatives should offer to provide the rest of the money that is needed?

	Frequency	*% of respondents*
Yes	512	52.4
No	325	33.2
Depends	138	14.1
Don't know/NA	3	0.3
Total	978	100.0

Consensus baseline: 75%

10b. (Respondents who said that relatives should not pay were asked this open-ended question. Up to three answers were post-coded.)
Why do you think that relatives should not be asked to pay part of the nursing home costs?

	Frequency	*% of responses*
Government/welfare state/ 'society' should pay	177	46
Relatives have other demands on their money	104	27
Relatives have no obligation	49	13
Private homes are too expensive	22	6
Old people want to be/should be independent	17	4
Other reason	15	4
Total	384	100

Consensus baseline: not applicable

11a. Suppose an elderly couple need to redecorate their home.
Do you think that relatives should offer to pay to have the work done?

	Frequency	*% of respondents*
Yes	538	55.0
No	342	35.0
Depends	98	10.0
Total	978	100.0

Consensus baseline: 75%

11b. (Respondents who said that relatives should 'not offer'.)
If the elderly couple cannot do the decorating themselves, do you think that they should *ask* relatives for the money to have it done?

	Frequency	*% of respondents*
Yes	69	20.2
No	241	70.4
Depends	28	8.2
NA	4	1.2
Total	342	100.0

Consensus baseline: 75%

12. A couple with children aged 9 and 14 have been evicted because they could not pay their rent. They cannot get a council flat and cannot afford a private one. Should relatives offer to give them a home for the next six months or so?

	Frequency	*% of respondents*
Yes	639	65.3
No	216	22.1
Don't know/depends	123	12.6
Total	978	100.0

Consensus baseline: 75%

13. There is a woman with children aged 3 and 5 who has just left her husband because he is violent. Should she:

	Frequency	*% of respondents*
Rent a flat, either privately or from the council	693	70.9
Ask relatives for a home for the next six months or so	250	25.6
Other (specified)	29	3.0
Don't know/NA	6	0.5
Total	978	100.0

Consensus baseline: 75%

14. Suppose an elderly person needs help with shopping and a little help in the home. The elderly person has an adult niece and nephew who live nearby and no other relatives. Should the niece and nephew take over responsibility for the tasks, or should someone else?

	Frequency	*% of respondents*
Niece and nephew	669	68.4
Someone else	209	21.4
Don't know/depends	100	10.2
Total	978	100.0

Consensus baseline: 75%

15a. If an elderly person, who has become very frail and can only move around with help, can no longer live alone should he or she move into an old people's home or go and live with relatives?

	Frequency	*% of respondents*
Move into an old people's home	537	54.9
Live with relatives	268	27.4
Don't know/depends	173	17.7
Total	978	100.0

Consensus baseline: 75%

15b. (Respondents who said 'old people's home'.)
Are there any circumstances in which the elderly person should live with relatives?

	Frequency	*% of respondents*
Yes	272	50.7
No	264	49.2
Don't know	1	0.1
Total	537	100.0

Consensus baseline: 75%

Appendix C: Who does what for whom?

WHO DOES WHAT FOR WHOM?

This appendix summarises data from our qualitative study on types of assistance which are given and received in families. We interviewed eighty-eight people in total, forty-nine women and thirty-nine men. Appendix A gives details of of how these data were collected.

The summary given here is only a very sketchy outline of some of the main patterns which emerge from our interviews. Some readers will find it useful to have it set out in this way, others may not. We were not attempting to construct an accurate account of precisely who does what. In contrast with our survey, we did not ask people identical questions phrased in precisely the same way. Therefore the numbers which we give in the summaries below should be taken simply as guides to identifying experiences which were common or rare among our study population, rather than an accurate representation. There may, for example, have been experiences which people had forgotten about, or where they had forgotten the precise sequence of events which led to some help being given. We do not wish to impose a spurious accuracy on our data to which our methods do not lend themselves. However, we did think that it would be useful to indicate the *range* of experiences which our study population have had, and for this reason we have separated out categories of assistance and included them in full, even where we have only one example in each category.

These are summaries of the simplest possible sort and they are incomplete in the sense that we have only included lists of items where we felt that we had reasonable confidence in our numbers. We have much more data than appears in these lists but we do not think it appropriate to express it in numerical form. For example, in relation to looking after children, we felt that we could say with a reasonable degree of certainly who was providing this type of assistance. We are less sure about whether we collected accurate information from everyone about the circumstances under which such assistance was provided, though we do have interesting data on this from some people. So read alone, these lists raise more questions than they answer. The discussion contained within the book chapters makes much more extensive use of the data in different ways.

In using these tables readers should note:

1 In most cases we have counted in the number of *examples* which we were given. Some interviewees gave us several under one heading, others might not have given us any.
2 In most cases, we have counted only those examples where the interviewee her/himself was involved. Where we have included 'third party' examples, we have stated that. This means that the interviewee reported an example which did not involve themselves directly, but concerned other people in their kin group.
3 The total number of people in our study population was eighty-eight.

1: Financial assistance

a. How many people have experience (either as donor or recipient) of giving or lending money within families?

Some experience reported:	women	45
	men	37
Interviewee indicated disapproval of giving/lending money in families:	women	2
No experience reported, but no expression of disapproval:	women	2
	men	2

b. For what purpose is money given/lent, and to whom?
Note: about 10 per cent of these examples concern third parties.

i. Daily living expenses (mostly small amounts of money):

Parent(s) to daughter	22
Parent(s) to son	12
Daughter to parent(s)	4
Son to parent(s)	3
Grandparent(s) to grand-daughter	5
Grandparent(s) to grandson	3
Sister to sister	2
Brother to brother	4
Sister to brother	2
Brother to sister	2
Regular sharing between groups of siblings	2

ii. Unemployment – help with living expenses:

Parents to son and wife	3
Mother to daughter and husband	1
Sister to brother	2

iii. Help with housing:

Parents to daughter (or daughter and husband)	13
Parents to son (or son and wife)	10
Sister to sister	1
Son to parents	1
Various relatives, presented as characteristic of Asian kin groups	2

iv. Education:

Parents to daughter	5
Parents to son	6
Aunt to niece	1
Brother to younger brother	1
Brother to younger sister	1
Grandmother to grandson	1

v. Employment (e.g. setting up a business):

Parents to daughter (or daughter and husband)	3
Parents to son (or son and wife)	5
Various relatives, presented as characteristic of Asian kin groups	2

vi. Migration:

Help given to assist a man's migration	3
Money sent to relatives overseas from people who had migrated to UK	2

vii. Other travel (leisure):

Parents to daughter	3
Parents to son	5
Grandmother to grandson	1
Son to mother	2
All relatives when visiting, according to Asian custom	1

viii. Payment for legal proceedings:

Father to daughter	1
Mother-in-law to son-in-law	1
Uncle to nephew	1

c. Daily living expenses: is the money a gift or a loan?

Parent(s) to daughter	
gift	15
loan	9
Parent(s) to son	
gift	8
loan	4
Daughter to parent(s)	
gift	2
loan	2
Son to parent(s)	
gift	2
loan	1
Grandparent(s) to grand-daughter	
gift	5
loan	0
Grandparent(s) to grandson	
gift	3
loan	0
Sister to sister	
gift	1
loan	1
Brother to brother	
gift	3
loan	1
Sister to brother	
gift	2
loan	0
Brother to sister	
gift	1
loan	1

2: Providing a home for a relative, either temporarily or permanently

a. Under what circumstances do adults live with a relative (other than their spouse and their immature children)?

Note:

Current examples = arrangements in the interviewee's own household at the time of interview.

Past examples = arrangements in which our interviewees have themselves been involved in the past, either as donor or recipient.

i. Young adults (under age 25) who have never left the parental home:

Current examples:	
Daughter	5
Son	5

Past examples not applicable

---

ii. Young adults who have left and returned (including students who are away in term time):

Current examples:	
Daughter	7
Son	4
Past examples:	
Son	1

---

iii. Never-married older people who have remained in the home of a parent:

Current examples:	
Son	1
Past examples:	
Son	3

---

iv. Married or cohabiting couples (not elderly) living with relatives, usually temporarily:

Current examples:	
With woman's parents	1
With man's parents	2
Past examples:	
With woman's parents	7
With man's parents	5
With woman's grandmother	2
With woman's sister	2

---

v. Divorced/separated/widowed people (not elderly) living with relatives:

Current examples	0
Past examples:	
Woman with her parents	5
Man with his parents	3
Brother with sister	2
Sister with brother	1

vi. Temporary sharing between two households which are normally separate:

Current examples:	
Man's mother as occasional temporary resident to help her financially	1
Past examples:	
Sharing between siblings' households while waiting for house to be available	1

vii. Elderly people sharing a home with a relative on a permanent basis:

Current examples:	
Mother / daughter's household	1
Mother / son's household	3
Past examples:	
Mother / daughter's household	2
Mother / son's household	3
Father / daughter's household	2

viii. Elderly people sharing a home with a relative on a short-term basis:

Current examples:	
Father / daughter's household	1
Past examples:	
Mother / daughter's household	1
Parents / son's household	1
Mother and stepfather / son's household	1
Father / son (staying in father's house)	1
Father / alternately in son's and daughter's household	1

b. How many people have experience of living in a household which contains an adult relative (categories ii–viii above)?

Have experienced this at some time in their lives:	
Women	28
Men	24
No such experience reported to us:	
Women	20
Men	16

3: Looking after young children

Note:

Regular arrangement = where an interviewee said that this is something which happens, or happened in the past, as part of a common pattern. It does not necessarily mean frequent.

Occasional arrangement = where interviewee cited specific individual occasions on which child care had been provided.

a. Who looks after whose children?

Mother's mother: regular	14
Mother's mother: occasional	5
Father's mother: regular	6
Father's mother: occasional	3
Mother's stepfather: regular	1
Mother's father: occasional	1
Father's sister: regular	1
Mother's brother: regular	1
Sisters looking after each other's children: occasional	5
Sister/brothers-in-law looking after each other's children: regular	1
Sisters-in-law looking after each other's children: occasional	3
Child's older sister and brother: regular	2
Child's older sister: occasional	1
Mother's aunt: occasional	1

b. If arrangement was regular, was any payment involved?

Payment to child's older siblings	2
Payment to maternal grandmother	1
No payment reported to us	22

4: Practical help

Who helps whom with practical tasks?

Note:

We asked open-ended questions about help with practical tasks, but did not itemise tasks separately. The examples here are those which our interviewees thought sufficiently important to mention.

i. Shopping:

Daughter for father	1
Son for father	1
Teenage daughter for parents – for payment	1
Daughter-in-law for mother-in-law	1

Grand-daughter for grandfather	2
Sister for sister	1
Brother for sister	2
Niece for uncle	1

ii. Cleaning in the house:

Daughter for mother	1
Young adult daughter in parental household	2
Young adult son in parental household cleaning own room	1
Daughter-in-law/mother-in-law cooperation in a shared household	1
Brother for sister	1
Cousin for cousin	1

iii. Cooking food:

Daughter for parents	1
Young adult daughter in parental household cooking own food	1
Mother for daughter and household	1
Mother for son and household	2
Father for daughter and household	1
Daughter-in-law/Mother-in-law cooperation in a shared household	2
Females cousins cooking communally-harvested produce	1
Aunt for nephew plus household	1

iv. Setting table and/or washing up dishes:

Young adult son in parental household	2

v. Washing and/or ironing clothes

Daughter for parents	1
Daughter for mother	1
Daughter for father	1
Young adult daughter in parental household doing own washing etc.	3
Daughter-in-law for mother-in-law	2
Grand-daughter for grandfather	1
Mother for daughter	2

vi. Looking after household while woman having a baby:

Parents for daughter	1

vii. Fitting plugs, other small electrical jobs:

Daughter, plus cohabitee, for mother	1
Nephew for aunt	1

viii. Gardening:

Daughter, plus cohabitee, for mother	1
Son for parent(s)	1
Grandson for grandfather	1
Nephew for aunt	1

ix. Sewing:

Female cousin for female cousin	2

x. House repairs and decoration, major assistance:

Daughter (or daughter plus husband) for mother	2
Son for parents	1
Father for daughter	1
Brother for sister	1
Uncle for niece	1
Male cousin for female cousin	1

xi. House repairs and decorations, limited assistance:

Daughter to mother	1
Son to mother	1
Father to daughter	2
Brother to sister	3

xii. Lifts in car:

Daughter to mother	1
Son to mother	2
Son to father	1
Daughter-in-law to parents-in-law	2
Father-in-law to daughter-in-law	1
Brother to sister	1
Brother-in-law to to sister-in-law	1
Nephew to aunt/uncle	2
Male cousin to cousin(s)	1

5: Caring for someone who is ill or incapacitated

Note:

i. *Major commitment* = where the person named was acting as the main supporter and/or where the time involved made a significant impact on daily life.

ii. In these tables the first number given represents examples where our interviewee her/himself had been involved as either donor or recipient. The number given in brackets represents third party examples.

a. Looking after relatives who are elderly: who looks after whom?

i. Long-term: major commitment

Daughter to mother	3	(11)
Daughter to father	3	(3)
Son to mother	2	(2)
Son to father	1	(0)
Daughter-in-law to mother-in-law	1	(4)
Daughter-in-law to father-in-law	1	(0)
Son-in-law to mother-in-law	1	(1)
Grandson to grandmother	2	(0)
Sister to sister	0	(1)
Brother to sister	1	(0)
Sister-in-law to husband's sister	1	(0)
Niece to aunt	1	(1)

ii. Short-term: major commitment

Daughter to mother	4	(5)
Daughter to father	0	(3)
Son to father	1	(2)
Daughter-in-law to mother-in-law	1	(1)
Daughter-in-law to father-in-law	1	(1)
Sister to sister	1	(0)
Sister to brother	1	(0)
Sister to brother's mother-in-law	1	(0)
Niece to aunt	2	(0)
Niece to uncle	1	(0)
Niece-in-law to husband's aunt	0	(1)

iii. Long-term: less significant commitment

Daughter to mother	4	(5)
Daughter to father	4	(0)
Son to mother	3	(3)
Son to father	2	(2)
Daughter-in-law to mother-in-law	3	(1)
Daughter-in-law to father-in-law	1	(0)
Son-in-law to mother-in-law	0	(1)
Son-in-law to father-in-law	2	(1)
Grand-daughter to grandmother	1	(0)
Grand-daughter to grandfather	1	(0)
Grand-daughter-in-law to husband's grandmother	1	(0)

iv. Short-term: less significant commitment

Daughter to mother	3	(0)
Daughter to father	3	(0)
Son to mother	1	(0)
Daughter-in-law to mother-in-law	1	(0)
Woman to cohabitee's mother	1	(0)
Son-in-law to mother-in-law	1	(0)
Grand-daughter to grandmother	1	(0)
Grandson to grandmother	1	(0)
Grandson to grandfather	2	(0)
Niece to aunt	3	(2)
Great nephew-in-law to wife's great aunt	1	(0)

b. Looking after adult relatives who are *not* elderly: who looks after whom?

i. Long-term: major commitment

Mother to daughter	0	(1)
Father to daughter	0	(1)
Parents to daughter	0	(1)
Sister to brother	0	(1)

ii. Short-term: major commitment

Daughter to father	1	(1)
Son to mother	1	(2)
Mother to son	1	(0)
Grandmother to grand-daughter	1	(0)

iii. Long-term: less significant commitment

Daughter to father	1	(0)

iv. Short-term: less significant commitment

Son to father	2	(1)
Son to mother	1	(0)
Mother to daughter	0	(1)
Parents to son	1	(1)
Mother-in-law to son-in-law	1	(0)
Sister to sister	0	(1)
Sister to brother	1	(0)
Brother to sister	2	(0)
Sister-in-law to sister's husband	0	(1)

c. Who reports looking after a relative (in any of the above categories)?

Reporting giving help:	women	24
	men	13
Reporting receiving help:	women	2
	men	3
Reporting giving and receiving:	women	3
	men	1
No mention of being involved in looking after/being looked after by a relative:	women	20
	men	22

6: Giving emotional support

Note: Examples here represent situations where someone helps someone else by listening, talking, giving advice.

Under what circumstances do people receive emotional support from relatives, and who gives it?

i. Divorce and separation: own

Mother to son	1
Parents-in-law to daughter-in-law	1
Parents-in-law to son-in-law	1
Parents to daughter	1
Parents to son	1
Brother to sister	1
Brother to brother	1

Brother to brother	1
Sister-in-law to brother-in-law	1
Female cousin to female cousin	1

ii. Divorce/separation of a close relative

| Daughter to parents | 1 |

iii. End of relationship with boy/girlfriend

Mother to son	1
Sister to sister	1
Sister to brother	1
Brother to sister	2
Aunt and uncle to nephew	1

iv. Bereavement

Daughter to mother	1
Daughter to father	1
Son to mother	3
Son to father	1
Son-in-law to father-in-law	1
Mother to daughter	2
Mother to son	2
Sister to sister	2
Sister to brother	1
Various cousins to female cousin	1

v. Serious illness of child

| Mother to daughter | 2 |
| Mother-in-law to son-in-law | 1 |

vi. Illness of close relative

Daughter to mother	1
Brother to sister	1
Brother to brother	2
Brother-in-law to sister's husband	1
Female cousin to female cousin	1

vii. Sexual problems

Mother to daughter	2
Female cousin to female cousin	1

viii. Problems at work

Parents to daughter	2
Female cousin to young male cousin	1

ix. Settling into new home after moving long distance

Parents to daughter	1
Sister to sister	1
Brother to brother	1

x. Having a baby

Mother to daughter	1

xi. Regular 'moral support' in a range of different circumstances

Daughter to mother	3
Son to mother	2
Mother to daughter	8
Mother to son	1
Father to daughter	1
Parents to daughter	4
Parents to son	4
Sister to sister	6
Sister to brother	3
Brother to sister	3
Brother to brother	5
Uncle to nephew	1
Female cousin to female cousin	2
'All the family'	3

References

Allan, G. (1985) *Family Life: Domestic Roles and Social Organization*, Oxford, Blackwell.

Allan, G. (1988) 'Kinship responsibility and care for elderly people', *Ageing and Society* 8: 249–68.

Anderson, D. (1990) 'The state of the social policy debate', in N. Manning and C. Ungerson (eds) *Social Policy Review 1989–90*, London, Longman.

Arber, S. and Gilbert, N. (1989) 'Men: the forgotten carers', *Sociology* 23 (1), 111–18.

Arber, S., Gilbert, N. and Evandrou, M. (1988) 'Gender, household composition and receipt of domiciliary services by elderly disabled people', *Journal of Social Policy* 17 (2), 153–75.

Becker, H.S. (1960) 'Notes on the concept of commitment', *American Journal of Sociology* 66: 32–40.

Bell, C. (1968) *Middle-class Families*, London, Routledge & Kegan Paul.

Bloch, M. (1973) 'The Long term and the short term: the economics and political significance of the morality of kinship.', in J. Goody (ed.) *The Character of Kinship*, Cambridge, Cambridge University Press.

Brannen, J. and Wilson, G. (1987) *Give and Take in Families*, London, Allen & Unwin.

Cheal, D. (1987) ' "Showing them you love them": gift giving and the dialectic of intimacy', *Sociological Review* 35: 150–69.

Cheal, D. (1988) *The Gift Economy*, London, Routledge.

Corrigan, P. (1989) 'Gender and the gift: the case of the family clothing economy', *Sociology* 23 (4), 515–34.

Crowther, M.A. (1982) 'Family responsibility and state responsibility in Britain before the Welfare State', *Historical Journal* 25 (1), 131–45.

Finch, J. (1987a) 'The vignette technique in survey research', *Sociology* 21 (1), 105–14.

Finch, J. (1987b) 'Family obligations and the life course', in A. Bryman, B. Bytheway, P. Allatt and T. Keil (eds) *Rethinking the Life Cycle*, London, Macmillan.

Finch, J. (1989) *Family Obligations and Social Change*, London, Polity.

Finch, J. (1990) 'The politics of community care in Britain', in C. Ungerson (ed.) *Gender and Caring: Work and Welfare in Britain and Scandinavia*, Hemel Hempstead, Harvester Wheatsheaf.

Finch, J. and Groves, D. (1980) 'Community care and the family: a case for equal opportunities?', *Journal of Social Policy* 9 (4), 487–514.

Finch, J. and Mason, J. (1990a) 'Decision-taking in the fieldwork process', in R.G. Burgess (ed.) *Studies in Qualitative Methodology*, London, JAI Press.

Finch, J. and Mason, J. (1990b) 'Filial obligations and kin support for elderly people', *Ageing and Society* 10: 151–75.

Finch, J. and Mason, J. (1990c) 'Divorce, remarriage and family obligations', *Sociological Review* 38 (2), 219–46.

Finch, J. and Mason, J. (1990d) 'Gender, employment and responsibilities to kin', *Work Employment and Society* 4 (3), 349–67.

Finch, J. and Mason, J. (1991) 'Obligations of kinship in contemporary Britain: is there normative agreement?', *British Journal of Sociology* 42 (3), 345–67.

Firth, R., Hubert, J. and Forge, A. (1970) *Families and their Relatives*, London, Routledge & Kegan Paul.

Fletcher, R. (1966) *The Family and Marriage in Britain*, Harmondsworth, Penguin.

Fortes, M. (1969) *Kinship and the Social Order*, Chicago, Aldine.

Goffman, E. (1967) *Interaction Ritual: Essays on Face-to-Face Behaviour*, New York, Anchor Books.

Gouldner, A.W. (1973) *For Sociology: Renewal and Critique in Sociology Today*, London, Allen Lane.

Green, H. (1988) *Informal Carers*, London, OPCS, HMSO.

Grieco, M. (1987) *Keeping it in the Family: Social Networks and Employment Change*, London, Tavistock.

Harris, N. (1988) 'Social security and the transition to adulthood', *Journal of Social Policy* 17 (4), 501–24.

Henwood, M. and Wicks, M. (1985) 'Community care, family trends and social change', *Quarterly Journal of Social Affairs* 1 (4), 357–71.

Leach, E.R. (1961) *Pul Eliya: A Village in Ceylon*, Cambridge, Cambridge University Press.

Lévi-Strauss, C. (1969) *The Elementary Structure of Kinship*, Boston, Beacon Press.

Macfarlane, A. (1978) *The Origins of English Individualism: The Family, Property and Social Transition*, Oxford, Blackwell.

Martin, J. and Roberts, C. (1984) *Women and Employment: a Lifetime Perspective*, Social Survey Division/OPCS, London, HMSO.

Mauss, M. (1954) *The Gift*, London, Cohen & West Ltd. (First published in France in 1950.)

Morgan, D.H.J. (1975) *Social Theory and the Family*, London, Routledge & Kegan Paul.

Morgan, D.H.J. (1985) *The Family, Politics and Social Theory*, London, Routledge & Kegan Paul.

Morris, L. (1990) *The Workings of the Household*, Cambridge, Polity.

Office of Population Censuses and Surveys (1982) *Census 1981 County Report: Greater Manchester*, Part I. London, HMSO.

Office of Population Censuses and Surveys (1983) *Census 1981 Sex, Age and Marital Status in Great Britain*, London, HMSO.

Office of Population Censuses and Surveys, Social Survey Division (1987) *General Household Survey 1985*, London, HMSO.

Parker, H. (1986) 'Family income support: government subversion of the traditional family', in D. Anderson and G. Dawson (eds) *Family Portraits*, London, Social Affairs Unit.

Quadagno, J. (1982) *Aging in Early Industrial Society: Work, Family and Social Policy in Nineteenth-century England*, London, Academic Press.

Qureshi, H. and Walker, A. (1989) *The Caring Relationship: Elderly People and their Families*, Basingstoke, Macmillan.

Rosser, C. and Harris, C.C. (1968) *The Family and Social Change*, London, Routledge & Kegan Paul.

Sahlins, M. (1965) 'On the sociology of primitive exchange', in M. Branton (ed.) *The Relevance of Models in Social Anthropology*, London, Tavistock.

Stacey, M. (1960) *Tradition and Change: A Study of Banbury*, Oxford, Oxford University Press.

Townsend, P. (1965) 'The effects of family structure on the likelihood of admission to an institution in old age: an application of general theory', in E. Shanas and G.F. Streib (eds) *Social Structure and the Family: Generational Relations*, Englewood Cliffs, NJ, Prentice Hall.

Ungerson, C. (ed.) (1990) *Gender and Caring: Work and Welfare in Britain and Scandinavia*, Hemel Hempstead, Harvester Wheatsheaf.

Wall, R. (1977) 'The responsibilities of kin', *Local Population Studies* 19: 58–60.

Wall, R. (1989) 'The living arrangements of the elderly in Europe in the 1980s', in B. Bytheway, T. Keil, P. Allatt and A. Bryman (eds) *Becoming and Being Old*, London, Sage.

Wallace, C. (1987) *For Richer for Poorer: Growing Up In and Out of Work*, London, Longman.

Wenger, G.C. (1984) *The Supportive Network*, London, Allen & Unwin.

Willmott, P. and Young, M. (1960) *Family and Class in a London Surburb*, London, Routledge & Kegan Paul.

Worsley, P. (1956) 'The kinship system of the Tallensi: a re-evaluation', *Journal of the Royal Anthropological Institute* 86: 37–75.

Young, M. and Willmott, P. (1957) *Family and Kinship in East London*, London, Routledge & Kegan Paul.

Name index

Subject index